The Easy KETO DIET COOKBOOK For Beginners

~ 2000+ ~

Days of Delicious and Easy to Cook Low-Carb Recipes to Fully Enjoy Your Ketogenic Diet

Elisa J. Williams

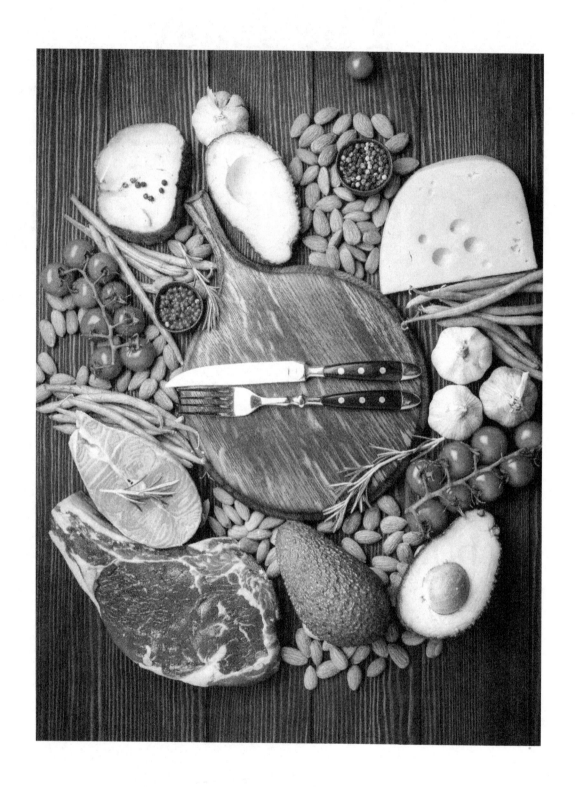

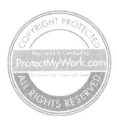

© Copyright 2023 by Elisa Williams - All rights reserved.

This includes backups in digital form. This concept is not limited to more classic forms of expression; it may be used to modern forms of expression as well, including digital ones.
In no event will the author or publisher be responsible for any losses incurred as a direct consequence of following the advice given in this book. It is possible to incur losses like these as a direct consequence of implementing the strategies outlined in this book. Nothing in this disclaimer will be construed to exclude liability for consequential, incidental, special, or punitive damages of any kind. There might be a direct or indirect link between the two, depending on the specifics of the situation.

Legal Notice:
This content can't be copied, duplicated, or sent in any way, either electronically or on paper, unless the author gives his or her written permission first. This publication can't be saved or recorded in any way, before or after the fact, without the publisher's permission. There has been no infringement on intellectual property rights.

Disclaimer Notice:

The information in this book has been carefully looked over and put together. On the other hand, there is no guarantee or warranty of any kind that the information is complete, correct, or useful.

If a reader chooses to act in a way that isn't helpful or makes a mistake, they won't be held responsible for any damage that happens as a result. You can't know for sure that you'll be successful. Because of this, the author doesn't take any responsibility for the fact that the book didn't meet the goals set out in the beginning.

TABLE OF CONTENTS

INTRODUCTION 1

BREAKFAST RECIPES 2
1. Breakfast Granola 2
2. Green Smoothie 2
3. Muffins Breakfast 3
4. Special Burrito 3
5. Coconut and Almonds Granola 3
6. Vegetarian Keto Breakfast Frittata 4
7. Mint Watermelon Bowl 4
8. Roasted Peppers Muffins 4
9. Tomato and Avocado Pizza 5
10. Sweet Cauliflower Rice Casserole 5
11. Breakfast Waffles 5
12. Nuts Porridge 6
13. Italian Scrambled Eggs 6
14. Healthy Keto Pancakes 6
15. Blueberry Soufflé 7
16. Classic French Toasts 7
17. Soy Chorizo, Eggs & Feta Cheese Plate 8
18. Spinach Omelet 8
19. Granola Breakfast Pops 9
20. Parsley Spread 9

VEGETARIAN MAINS 10
21. Avocado and Kale Soup 10
22. Creamy Brussels Sprouts Bowls 10
23. Green Beans and Radishes Bake 11
24. Avocado and Radish Bowls 11
25. Celery and Radish Soup 11
26. Lime Avocado and Cucumber Soup 12
27. Grilled Veggie Mix 12
28. Spinach and Cucumber Salad 12
29. Curry Spinach Soup 13
30. Arugula and Artichokes Bowls 13
31. Keto Tofu and Spinach Casserole 13
32. Low-Carb Jambalaya 13
33. Chili-Garlic Edamame 14
34. Eggplant Pomodoro 14
35. Vietnamese "Vermicelli" Salad 14
36. Homemade Vegan Sausages 15
37. Avocado, Endive and Asparagus Mix 15
38. Collard Greens and Garlic Mix 15
39. Seitan Cauliflower Bowl 16
40. Arugula Tomato Salad 16

SOUPS AND STEWS 17
41. Beef Stew 17
42. Turkey Soup 18
43. Tomato and Basil Soup 18
44. Chicken and Mushroom Soup 19
45. Coconut Chicken Soup 19
46. Lemon Soup 19
47. Black Bean Soup 20
48. Creamy Garlic-Spinach Rotini Soup 20
49. White and Wild Mushroom Barley Soup 21
50. Italian Wedding Soup 21
51. Spinach and Watermelon Soup 22
52. Broccoli Soup 22
53. Hot & Sour Tofu Soup 22
54. Autumn Medley Stew 23
55. Tuscan White Bean Soup 23
56. Mexican Fideo Soup with Pinto Beans 24
57. Lamb and Coconut Stew 24
58. Veggie and Kale Stew 25
59. Lemony Lentil and Rice Soup 25
60. Roasted Vegetable Bisque 26

SALADS RECIPE 27
61. Mango salad 27
62. Shrimp and Asparagus Salad 28
63. Carrot and walnut salad 28
64. Pickled onion salad 28
65. Strawberries and Avocado Salad 28
66. Pickled Grape Salad with Pear, Taleggio, and Walnuts 29
67. Fresh Fruit Salad 29
68. Dried apricot sauce 29
69. Tomato, Cucumber, and Basil Salad 30
70. Caramelized Onion and Beet Salad 30
71. Spinach Salad With Orange-Dijon Dressing 31
72. Golden Couscous Salad 31
73. Quinoa Salad with Black Beans And Tomatoes 31
74. Caesar Salad 32
75. Classic Potato Salad 32
76. Black Bean Taco Salad Bowl 33
77. Tuna Caprese Salad 33
78. Chopped Salad 34
79. Moroccan Aubergine Salad 34
80. Warm Lentil Salad with Red Wine Vinaigrette .35

FISH & SEAFOOD 36
81. Fish Tacos 36
82. Paleo Salmon 37
83. Fish Dish 37
84. Salmon Skewers 37
85. Shrimp Dish 38
86. Grilled Hake 38
87. Coconut Pollock 39
88. Spicy Paella 39
89. Fish Cakes with Greens 39
90. Fish Bars 40
91. Tuna Pie 40
92. Grilled Calamari 41

93.	Scallops, Grapes and Spinach Bowls	41
94.	Spanish Mussels	41
95.	Tilapia Broccoli Platter	42
96.	Halibut And Tasty Salsa	42
97.	Light Lobster Bisque	43
98.	Thai Pumpkin Seafood Stew	43
99.	Herbal Shrimp Risotto	43
100.	Mackerel and Orange Medley	44

BEEF, PORK, POULTRY & LAMB 45

101.	Beef Teriyaki	45
102.	Chicken with Bok Choy	46
103.	Beef Skillet	46
104.	Pork With Pear Salsa	46
105.	Chicken with Sprouts and Beets	47
106.	Chicken with Grapes	47
107.	Pork Tenderloin with Carrot Puree	47
108.	Pork with Strawberry Sauce	48
109.	Moroccan Lamb	48
110.	Roasted Lamb	49
111.	Beef Casserole	49
112.	Grilled Lamb Chops	50
113.	Lamb Casserole	50
114.	Lamb Chops with Mint Sauce	50
115.	Pork with Blueberry Sauce	51
116.	Chili Turkey and Peppers	51
117.	Pulled Pork	52
118.	Turkey with Tomato Asparagus	52
119.	Beef And Wonderful Gravy	52
120.	Sheppard's Pie	53

SNACKS 54

121.	Seeds Bowls	54
122.	Almond Artichoke Dip	54
123.	Snow Peas and Tomato Salsa	55
124.	Apple Chips	55
125.	Dill Cucumber Dip	55
126.	Beans Salsa	56
127.	Balsamic Mushrooms Mix	56
128.	Balsamic Pineapple Bites	56
129.	Parsley Pearl Onions Mix	56
130.	Keto Broccoli Sticks	57
131.	Nori Snack Rolls	57
132.	Risotto Bites	57
133.	Marinated Mushroom Wraps	58
134.	Curried Tofu "Egg Salad" Pitas	58
135.	Patch Garden Sandwiches	59
136.	Spinach Garlic Dip	59
137.	Sesame- Wonton Crisps	60

DESSERTS 61

138.	Cheesecake	61
139.	Low-Carb Chocolate Coconut Fat Bombs	62
140.	Crunchy Cherry Chocolate Confections	62
141.	Low-Carb Keto Caramels	63
142.	Coconut Chocolate Bars	63
143.	Almond-Date Energy Bites	63
144.	Keto Chocolate Mug Cake	64
145.	Keto Chocolate Chip Muffins	64
146.	Low-Carb, Keto Strawberry Fat Bombs	65
147.	Paleo Vegan Peppermint Patties	65
148.	Berries and Cherries Bowls	65
149.	Cocoa Peach Cream	66
150.	Nuts and Seeds Pudding	66
151.	Cashew Fudge	66
152.	Apple Crumble	66
153.	Apricots Cake	67
154.	Banana Chocolate Cupcakes	67
155.	Peach-Mango Crumble (Pressure cooker)	68

CONCLUSION 69

CONVERSION MEASUREMENT 70

INTRODUCTION

Do you want to make a change in your life?
Do you want to become a healthier person who can enjoy a new and improved life?
Then, you are definitely in the right place. You are about to discover a great and very healthy diet that has changed the lives of millions of people around the world. We are talking of the ketogenic diet, a lifestyle that will transform you into a new person in no time.

Essentially, a ketogenic diet is a diet that drastically restricts your carb intake and fat intake; this pushes your body to go into a state of ketosis.
Your body uses glucose from carbs to fuel metabolic pathways—meaning various bodily functions like digestion and breathing—essentially anything that needs energy. Glucose is, therefore, the primary pathway when it comes to sourcing the body's energy.
But the body also has another pathway, and it can make use of fats to fuel the various bodily processes. And this is what is called ketosis. The body can only enter ketosis when there is no glucose available, thus the reason why eating a low-carb diet is essential in the keto diet. Since no glucose is available, the body is pushed to use fats—it can either come from the food you consume or from your body's fat reserves—the adipose tissue or from the flabby parts of your body. This is how the keto diet helps you lose weight by burning up all those stored fats that you have and using them to fuel bodily processes.

Ketosis is a very natural process, the body will soon adapt to this state, and therefore you will be able to lose weight in no time, but you will also become healthier, and your physical and mental performances will improve. Your blood sugar levels will improve, and you won't be predisposed to diabetes. Also, epilepsy and heart disease can be easily prevented if you are on a ketogenic diet. Your cholesterol will improve, and you will feel amazing in no time. How does that sound?

Inside this cookbook, you will discover 1500 of the best Ketogenic recipes in the world, and you will soon be able to make each and every one of them easily at home. You will have enough recipes for a lifetime of keto meals.

But there's more. For those who want to stick to a Keto Vegetarian Diet Plan, more than 800 recipes are included in this cookbook!

I hope you'll like it and you will be able to use this cookbook to enjoy the benefits of the keto diet and transform your life. Enjoy!

BREAKFAST RECIPES

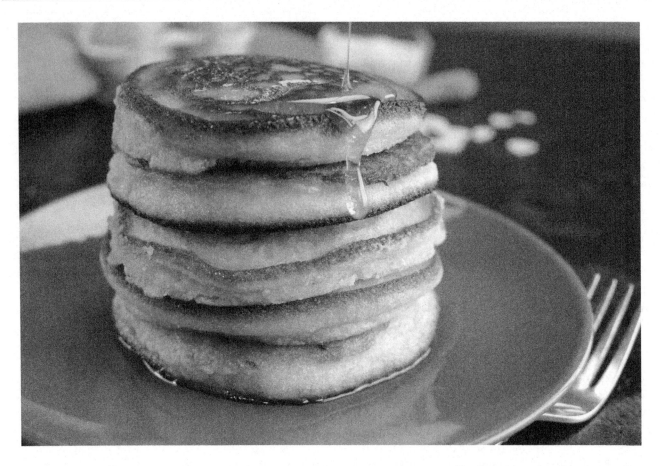

1. Breakfast Granola

Duration for preparing: 55 mins.
Persons: 6

Required Material:

- 10 gr cinnamon powder
- 180 gr almond flour
- 10 gr ground nutmeg
- 40 gr coconut flakes
- 10 ml vanilla extract
- 60 gr chopped walnuts
- 80 ml coconut oil
- 30 gr hemp hearts

Instructions:

1. Distribute on a baking tray after mixing almond flour, coconut flakes, cinnamon, nutmeg, vanilla, hemp, and walnuts together in a dish.
2. Oven-bake at 135 C (275 F) for 50 mins, stirring once every 10 mins.. Once the granola is cool, spoon it onto dishes and eat it for breakfast

Nutritional breakdown:
Calories: 393, Total Fat: 36g, Sodium: 4mg, Carbs: 14g, Fiber: 8g, Sugars: 2g, Protein: 10g

2. Green Smoothie

Duration for preparing: 5 mins.
Persons: 3

Required Material:

- 1 small cucumber; peeled and chopped
- 1 green apple; chopped
- Juice of 1/2 lemon

- Juice of 1/2 lime
- 5 gr ginger; finely grated
- 7 gr gelatin powder
- 65 gr kale; chopped
- 240 ml coconut water

Instructions:
1. Pulse the apple, cucumber, ginger, and kale together a few times in a food processor or blender.
2. Combine gelatin powder, lime and other lemon juice, and coconut water in a blender.
3. Instantly serve after pouring into glasses.

Nutritional breakdown:
Calories: 108, Total Fat: 2g, Sodium: 100mg, Carbs: 21g, Fiber: 5g, Sugars: 12g, Protein: 3g

3. Muffins Breakfast

Duration for preparing: 40 mins.
Persons: 4

Required Material:
- 65 gr kale; chopped
- Some coconut oil for greasing the muffin cups
- 10 gr chives; finely chopped
- 120 ml almond milk
- 6 eggs
- Black pepper

Instructions:
1. Beat the eggs with the chives and the kale in the dish.
2. Incorporate some grains of black pepper into the almond milk for flavor. Distribute the batter evenly among 8 greased muffin cups.
3. Insert in an already-heated oven at a temperature of 175 °C (350 °F). Cook for 30 mins.. The best way to enjoy freshly baked muffins is to serve them warm, right out of the oven after a brief cooling period.

Nutritional breakdown:
Calories: 148, Fat: 11g, Cholesterol: 279mg, Sodium: 97mg, Carbs: 3g, Fiber: 1g, Sugars: 1g, Protein: 9g

4. Special Burrito

Duration for preparing: 25 mins.
Persons: 2

Required Material:
- 60 gr canned green chilies; chopped
- One small chopped yellow onion
- 4 eggs; egg yolks and whites divided
- 60 gr cilantro
- A red sweet pepper
- 2 tomatoes; chopped
- 113 gr beef; ground and brown for 10 mins.
- 1 avocado; peeled, pitted, and chopped
- Some hot sauce for serving
- A drizzle of Oil of olive

Instructions:
1. Put a little Oil of olive in a pan over a moderately high flame. After whisking the egg whites in a bowl, lay half of them out evenly, and cook for 1 minute.
2. Cook for a further minute after flipping, then transfer to a dish and repeat with the remaining egg whites.
3. To the same pan, add the onions and cook for 1 minute while stirring occasionally.
4. Toss in the chilies, peppers, tomatoes, meat, and cilantro for 5 mins., stirring occasionally. Incorporate in egg yolks and continue cooking till they are set.
5. Distribute the egg and meat mixture between two egg-white tortillas, sprinkle with the avocado and spicy sauce, and wrap up to serve for breakfast.

Nutritional breakdown:
Calories: 497, Fat: 36g, Cholesterol: 357mg, Sodium: 226mg, Carbs: 20g, Fiber: 8g, Sugars: 6g, Protein: 27g

5. Coconut and Almonds Granola

Duration for preparing: 45 mins.
Persons: 4

Required Material:
- 225g coconut flakes
- 180g chopped almonds
- 80g sesame seeds

- 80g sunflower seeds
- 2.5g ground cinnamon
- 15ml chia seeds
- 120ml maple syrup
- A pinch of cardamom
- 30ml vanilla extract
- 2 tbsp Oil of olive

Instructions:
1. In the dish, include the almonds, sunflower seeds, roasted sesame seeds, coconut, chia seeds, cardamom, and cinnamon and mix well.
2. In the meanwhile, bring the oil, vanilla extract, and maple syrup to a boil in a small saucepan at a heat range between low and medium for around one minute while stirring constantly.
3. After pouring this mixture over the almond mixture and swirling it to incorporate the two, spread the mixture out on a baking sheet and set the timer for 30 mins. at a temperature of 150 degrees Celsius.
4. Stir the mixture once at the 15-minute mark. Before serving, it is recommended to wait till your homemade granola has fully cooled down.

Nutritional breakdown:
Calories: 501, Fat: 42g, Sodium: 12mg, Carbs: 26g, Fiber: 12g, Sugars: 9g, Protein: 12g

6. Vegetarian Keto Breakfast Frittata

Duration for preparing: 10 mins.
Ready in: 5 mins.
Persons: 4

Required Material:
- 4 organic eggs
- 1.25g of sea salt
- 1 avocado, peeled, and sliced
- 60 grams of grated cheddar cheese
- 10 pitted olives
- 1.50g Herbes de Provence
- 30ml of Oil of olive
- 28 grams of butter

Instructions:
1. Beat together the Herb de Provence, eggs, olives, and salt till frothy, after adding to a mixing bowl.
2. Butter must be melted over low heat in a pan.
3. Put avocado slices in a hot pan and cook them till they start to become golden.
4. The eggs should be placed into the pan, and the cheese should be sprinkled on top, before being removed from the heat.
5. Cook for three mins. with the lid on, either at or slightly over the boiling point. Cook for a further two mins. after flipping.
6. Serve the frittata with sliced avocados on a plate and enjoy!

Nutritional Values for Serving:
Calories: 325, Fat: 28g, Carbs: 6g, Protein: 15g, Fiber: 3g, Net Carbs: 3g

7. Mint Watermelon Bowl

Duration for preparing: 5 mins.
Ready in: 0 mins.
Persons: 2

Required Material:
- 320 grams of watermelon, peeled and cut into cubes
- 6 pitted and sliced kalamata olives
- 5ml avocado oil
- ½ tablespoon (7.5 ml) of balsamic vinegar
- 15g of chopped fresh mint

Instructions:
1. Watermelon, olives, and other components may be tossed together in a dish, then served in individual portions.

Nutritional breakdown:
Calories: 85, Fat: 4g, Carbs: 12g, Protein: 2g, Fiber: 2g, Net Carbs: 11g

8. Roasted Peppers Muffins

Duration for preparing: 10 mins.
Ready in: 15 mins.
Persons: 6

Required Material:
- 18g of flax seeds mixed with 45ml of water
- 80 grams of chopped spinach
- 120ml of coconut cream
- 25 grams of grated cashew cheese
- 75 grams of roasted peppers, red
- A dash of salt and black pepper
- 6g of chopped fresh oregano
- 2g of chili powder
- Cooking spray

Instructions:
1. Using a whisk, incorporate all of the components that are required for the spinach combination, minus the cooking spray, in the dish.
2. Spoon the pepper combination into a prepared muffin tray, bake it in the oven at 200 degrees C for 15 mins., and then savor it for breakfast.

Nutritional breakdown:
Calories: 160, Fat: 13g, Carbs: 7g, Protein: 5g, Fiber: 3g, Net Carbs: 4g

9. Tomato and Avocado Pizza

Duration for preparing: 20 mins.
Ready in: 20 mins.
Persons: 2

Required Material:
- 240 grams of almond flour
- A pinch of salt and black pepper
- 355ml of water
- 30ml of avocado oil
- 1g granulated chili
- 1 tomato, sliced
- 1 avocado, peeled and sliced
- 60 gr of tomato puree
- 10g chopped fresh chives

Instructions:
1. Incorporate the flour, salt, pepper, water, oil, and chili granulate together in a large bowl. Lightly knead the dough, then set it aside for 20 mins. covered.
2. Roll out the dough into a circle on a floured surface, then set it in a baking tin lined. Cook for 10 mins. at 200 degrees C in an already-heated oven.
3. After laying the pizza dough on a baking sheet, put the tomato passata on top and the other ingredients.
4. Prepare some breakfast slices.

Nutritional breakdown:
Calories: 630, Fat: 54g, Carbs: 25g, Protein: 17g, Fiber: 12g, Net Carbs: 8g

10. Sweet Cauliflower Rice Casserole

Duration for preparing: 10 mins.
Ready in: 1 hour
Persons: 8

Required Material:
- 360 g of blackberries
- 240 g of coconut cream
- 5g of ground cinnamon
- 10ml of vanilla extract
- 2g ginger powder
- 240 grams of cauliflower rice
- 30 grams of chopped walnuts
- 480 ml of almond milk

Instructions:
1. Ingredients, including cauliflower rice, berries, cream, and the rest, should be incorporated in a tin and cooked at 175 degrees C for 60 mins.
2. Dish out the concoction for breakfast in separate servings.

Nutritional breakdown:
Calories per serving: 170, Fat: 13g, Carbs: 12g, Protein: 3g, Fiber: 4g, Net Carbs: 9g

11. Breakfast Waffles

Duration for preparing: 20 mins.
Persons: 4

Required Material:
- 2 eggs
- 120ml almond milk
- 30ml coconut oil; melted
- 1.2g; ground
- 12g baking powder

- 7g coconut flour
- 42g honey
- 180g almond flour
- 30g tapioca flour
- 7.5ml vanilla extract
- Pure maple syrup for serving

Instructions:
1. In the bowl of your mixer, stir together coconut flour, almond flour, tapioca flour, baking powder, and cinnamon.
2. Add egg, almond milk, coconut oil, honey, and vanilla extract, and mix very well.
3. In another bowl, use your mixer to whip the egg whites.
4. Add them to the waffle mix and stir it all very well.
5. Pour this mixture into your waffle iron to create 8 waffles.
6. Put them on plates, top them with maple syrup, and serve.

Nutritional breakdown:
Calories: 509; Fat: 41g; Fiber: 4g; Carbs: 24g; Protein: 13g

12. Nuts Porridge

Duration for preparing: 15 mins.
Persons: 2

Required Material:
- 60g pecans; soaked overnight and drained
- 1/2 banana; mashed
- 180ml hot water
- 30g coconut butter
- 1.2g cinnamon
- 10ml. maple syrup

Instructions:
1. In a blender, mix pecans with water, banana, coconut butter, cinnamon, and maple syrup, pulse really well, and transfer to a small pot.
2. Heat everything up over medium heat, cook till it's creamy, transfer to serving bowls, and serve.

Nutritional breakdown:
Calories: 426; Fat: 42.8g; Fiber: 5.5g; Carbs: 16.9g; Protein: 5.5g

13. Italian Scrambled Eggs

Duration for preparing: 10 mins.
Ready in: 10 mins.
Persons: 1

Required Material:
- 2 eggs, whisked
- 1.25g rosemary
- 120g cherry tomatoes halved
- 180g cups kale
- 2.5ml coconut oil, melted
- 45ml water
- 5ml balsamic vinegar
- ¼ avocado

Instructions:
1. The kale, rosemary, water and tomatoes go into oil that has been heated to a medium-low temperature. For about five mins., while stirring occasionally, cover the mixture.
2. After 4 mins., include the egg, give the mixture a swirl, and scramble it.
3. Put in some Balsamic vinegar, mix, and serve over avocado slices. Enjoy!

Nutritional breakdown:
Calories 345, Fat 25.3g, Fiber 6.1g, carbs 14.7g, protein 17.2g

14. Healthy Keto Pancakes

Duration for preparing: 10 mins.
Ready in: 2 mins.
Persons: 6

Required Material:
- 1 large banana, mashed
- 2 organic eggs
- 0.30g baking powder
- 20g vanilla protein powder

Instructions:
1. The ideal temperature range for pre-heating a skillet is between low and medium. Just throw everything into a dish and stir till combined. Apply nonstick cooking spray to the pan.
2. Put three tablespoons of batter into a very hot to make a pancake.

3. Cook the pancake for no more than one minute on one side before flipping it over to cook for another minute.
4. Eat with sugar-free syrup on top!

Nutritional breakdown:
Calories: 78 Fat: 1.6 g Carbohydrates: 5.5 g Sugar: 3 g Protein: 11.1 g Cholesterol: 55 mg

15. Blueberry Soufflé

Duration for preparing: 15 mins.
Ready in: 20 mins.
Serving: 4

Required Material:
For the blueberry sauce:
- 150g frozen blueberries
- 10g erythritol
- 15ml water

For the omelet:
- 4 egg yolks, room temperature
- 30g erythritol, divided
- 3 egg whites, room temperature
- 5ml Oil of olive
- ½ lemon, zested to garnish

Instructions:
For the blueberry sauce:
1. Pour the blueberries, erythritol, and water into a small casserole. Cook with occasional stirring till the berries soften and become syrupy, about 10 mins. Stir in the vanilla and cool slightly.

For the omelet:
2. Star your oven to 175°C.
3. Egg yolks and half erythritol should be whisked together before thick and pale in color in a large basin using an electric whisk. Egg whites should be whisked on a moderate speed with clean beaters til frothy in a separate basin. Once soft peaks form, which should take around 3–4 mins. if you increase the speed, add the other erythritol and whisk. Slowly incorporate the egg white mixture into the yolk mixture by folding it in.
4. Oil of olive should be heated in a pan that can go from stovetop to oven without sticking. Swirl the pan to evenly distribute the oil, then add the egg mixture and continue to stir while it cooks. Bake for 2–3 mins., till golden, puffed, and set, after cooking for 3 mins..
5. Serve the omelet with a dollop of blueberry sauce after put it on a plate, spread it with a spoon. Distribute some lemon zest on top.
6. Tea and coffee may be served right away together.

Nutritional breakdown:
Calories: 120, Total Fat: 7g, Fat: 7 g, Carbs: 8g, Fiber: 2g, Sugar: 5g, Protein: 8g

16. Classic French Toasts

Duration for preparing: 10 mins.
Ready in: 6 mins.
Serving: 6 mins.

Required Material:
For the glass dish bread:
- 16g flax seed meal + 90ml water
- 5g butter
- 16g coconut flour
- 16g almond flour
- 6g baking powder
- A pinch salt
- 30ml coconut cream

For the toast's batter:
- 16g flax seed meal + 90ml water
- 30ml coconut milk
- 0.5g cinnamon powder + extra for garnishing
- 1 pinch salt
- 30g butter

Instructions:
For the glass dish bread:
1. For the flax egg, whisk both quantities of flax seed powder with mixing water in two separate bowls and leave to soak for 5 mins..
2. Then, grease a glass dish (for the microwave) with the butter.
3. The coconut flour, almond flour, baking powder, and salt should all be combined in a separate basin.
4. Once the flax seed egg is done, incorporate the cream from the coconut with a part of it and then combine the resulting mixture with the rest of the dry components. Whip the

mixture continuously till there are no more lumps and it is completely slick.
5. Include the dough into the glass dish and microwave for 2 mins. or till the middle part of the bread is done.
6. Take out and allow the bread to cool. Then, remove the bread and slice in half. Return to the glass dish.

For the toast:
7. The extra flax egg, cinnamon, and salt should be whisked into the coconut cream.
8. Immerse the bread in the mixture overnight. Make sure all of the batter is soaked up by turning the bread over a few times.
9. Then, in a frying pan, soften the butter and cook the bread slices on both sides in the melted butter.
10. Once the bread is a deep golden color on both sides, take it from the pan and scatter it with the powdered cinnamon. Eat hot with tea or bulletproof coffee.

Nutritional breakdown:
Calories: 164, Total Fat: 14g, Total Carbs: 7g, Fiber: 4g, Sugar: 1g, Protein: 4g

17. Soy Chorizo, Eggs & Feta Cheese Plate

Duration for preparing: 10 mins.
Ready in: 5 mins.
Serving: 4

Required Material:
- 5ml Oil of olive
- 2.3g smoked paprika
- 85g soy chorizo, diced
- 4 eggs
- 120 g crumbled feta cheese
- 2 green onions, thinly sliced diagonally
- 6g fresh parsley
- Greek yogurt to serve

Instructions:
1. First, adjust your oven to 175 degrees C. In a saucepan with a level base that can go from stovetop to oven, combine the sunflower oil and paprika for 30 seconds. Lightly brown the soy chorizo in the pan, then transfer it to a dish and set aside the sunflower oil.
2. Following 2 mins., crack the eggs into the pan and put the chorizo and feta cheese on top, being sure not to touch the egg yolks.
3. Return the pan to the oven for another minute or two, so that the egg yolks are almost set but still a bit runny in the middle, at which point they may be garnished with green shallots and parsley. Greek yogurt is delicious when served warm.

Nutritional breakdown:
Calories: 209, Total fat: 14 g, Cholesterol: 217 mg, Sodium: 646 mg, Total carbohydrates: 3 g, Dietary fiber: 1 g, Sugar: 1 g, Protein: 18 g

18. Spinach Omelet

Duration for preparing: 10 mins.
Ready in: 15 mins.
Persons: 4

Required Material:
- 2 eggs, whisked
- 15ml ghee, melted
- A pinch of black pepper
- 30g baby spinach, torn
- 1 onion
- 5g thyme springs
- 3 garlic cloves
- 2 chopped sweet pepper, red and green
- 45ml oil of olive
- 250ml cherry tomatoes, halved
- 1 red chili pepper

Instructions:
1. Melt the ghee in a pan over a moderate flame. Eggs and a dash of black pepper are on the list. Keep stirring for around five mins. to ensure even cooking. Stir together, simmer for a further two to three mins., and then serve.
2. In another pan, heat the oil; after it is heated, add the shallots and cook them for three mins. while stirring them occasionally. Sprinkle the omelet with the garlic-thyme-tomato-red-yellow-and-chili pepper combination after 5 mins. of additional cooking time.
3. Hot breakfast should be prepared and served.

4. Enjoy!

Nutritional breakdown:
Calories: 186, Total fat: 16 g, Cholesterol: 163 mg Sodium: 77 mg, Total carbohydrates: 6 g, Dietary fiber: 2 g, Sugar: 3 g, Protein: 6 g

19. Granola Breakfast Pops

Duration for preparing: 5 mins
Persons: 4-6

Required Material:
- 80g chopped fresh pineapple
- 80g chopped mango
- 480ml. low fat vanilla yogurt
- 20g sugar free granola
- 75g chopped strawberries

Instructions:
1. In a mixing container, incorporate the yogurt with the chopped strawberries, pineapple, and mango. Combine thoroughly.
2. After transferring the yogurt batter to the ice pop forms, apply a little amount of granola into every one of the molds.
3. Put it in the freezer to chill and let it stay there for at least a few hours or all night.

Nutritional breakdown:
Calories: 108, Total fat: 2 g, Cholesterol: 7 mg, Sodium: 55 mg, Total carbohydrates: 17 g, Dietary fiber: 1 g, Sugar: 14 g, Protein: 7 g

20. Parsley Spread

Duration for preparing: 5 mins.
Ready in: 0 mins.
Persons: 8

Required Material:
- 60g parsley leaves
- 240ml coconut cream
- 10g sun-dried tomatoes
- 30ml lime juice
- 40g shallots
- 1g oregano
- A dash of salt, and some freshly powdered grains black pepper

Instructions:
1. After combining the parsley, cream, tomatoes, and all the other components in the bowl of a blender, blend the mixture well, divide the mixture into dishes and serving it for breakfast.

Nutritional breakdown:
Calories: 71, Total fat: 7 g, Sodium: 32 mg, Total carbohydrates: 2 g, Dietary fiber: 0 g, Sugar: 1 g, Protein: 1 g

VEGETARIAN MAINS

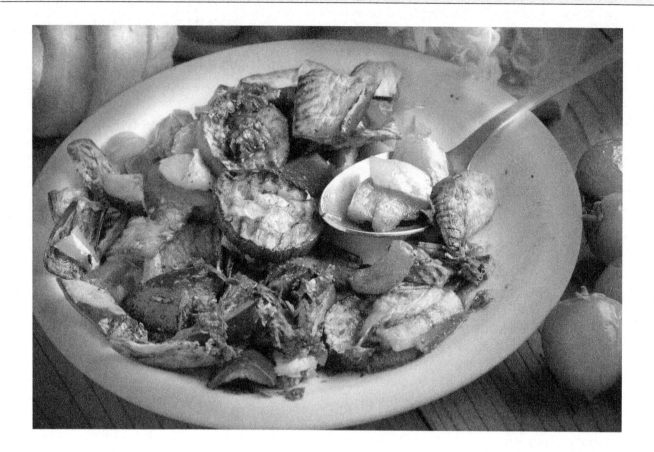

21. Avocado and Kale Soup

Duration for preparing: 5 mins.
Ready in: 7 mins.
Persons: 4

Required Material:

- 200 g curly kale, torn into pieces
- 5 g of turmeric powder
- 1 avocado, pitted, peeled, and sliced
- 1 liter of vegetable broth
- One Juice of lime
- 2 garlic
- 30g of chopped chives
- Salt & black pepper

Instructions:

1. After adding the kale and avocado to a pot and cooking it for seven mins. on a heat that is somewhere between low and medium, the mixture should be pureed using a hand-held blender, and then it should be divided among individual dishes for serving.

Nutritional breakdown:

Calories 105, Fat 7g, Fiber 5g, Carbs 11g, Protein 4g

22. Creamy Brussels Sprouts Bowls

Duration for preparing: 10 mins.
Ready in: 30 mins.
Persons: 4

Required Material:

- 15 ml of Oil of olive
- 450 g Brussels sprouts, cleaned and halved
- 240 ml of coconut cream
- 2g of chili granulate
- 2.5ml of garam masala

- 2.5g of garlic powder
- A pinch of salt and black pepper
- 15 ml of lime juice

Instructions:
1. In a roasting pan, combine the sprouts with the To prepare the sprouts, put them in a roasting pan along with the cream, chili granulates, and additional ingredients. Then, place the pan in an oven that has been warmed to 190 degrees Celsius for 30 mins..
2. Dish up in separate bowls as an appetizer or a light dinner.

Nutritional breakdown:
Calories: 235, Fat: 20g, Sodium: 68mg, Carbs: 12g, Fiber: 4g, Sugar: 3g, Protein: 4g.

23. Green Beans and Radishes Bake

Duration for preparing: 10 mins.
Ready in: 25 mins.
Persons: 4

Required Material:
- 15 ml Oil of olive
- 454 gr green beans, trimmed and halved
- 250 gr radishes, sliced
- 240 gr coconut cream
- 2g sweet paprika
- 120 gr cashew cheese, shredded
- A dash of salt, and some freshly powdered grains black pepper
- 15g chives

Instructions:
1. Throw the green beans, radishes, and the other ingredients, except the cheese, in a roasting pan and toss to combine.
2. After distributing the cheese on top, bake the dish for another 25 mins. at 190 degrees Celsius.
3. For presentation, distribute the mixture out into a suitable number of plates.

Nutritional breakdown:
Calories: 410, Fat: 34g, Sodium: 255mg, Carbs: 20g, Fiber: 6g, Sugar: 7g, Protein: 12g.

24. Avocado and Radish Bowls

Duration for preparing: 10 mins.
Ready in: 0 mins.
Persons: 4

Required Material:
- 475 gr radishes, halved
- 2 avocados, peeled, pitted, and roughly cubed
- 30 ml coconut cream
- 30 ml balsamic vinegar
- 15g green onion
- 2g chili powder
- 120 gr baby spinach
- A dash of salt, and some freshly powdered grains black pepper

Instructions:
1. In the dish, unite the radishes, avocados, and the other ingredients, mix everything together, and eat as a light meal.

Nutritional breakdown:
Calories: 215, Fat: 19g, Sodium: 81mg, Carbs: 13g, Fiber: 8g, Sugar: 3g, Protein: 3g.

25. Celery and Radish Soup

Duration for preparing: 10 mins.
Ready in: 20 mins.
Persons: 4

Required Material:
- 225 gr radishes, cut into quarters
- 2 celery stalks
- 30ml Oil of olive
- 4 scallions
- 5g fennel seeds, crushed
- 5g coriander
- 1,4 lt vegetable stock
- A dash of salt, and some freshly powdered grains black pepper
- 6 garlic cloves
- 15g chives

Instructions:
1. It is recommended that the garlic, onions, and celery be sautéed for about five mins. in the oil that is already warm in the pan.
2. Come all of the ingredients to a boil,

preserve for later the radishes, cover, and cook everything for 15 mins. at a temperature that is either a little below or barely above the point of the boil. To serve, divide the mixture evenly among separate bowls.

Nutritional breakdown:

Calories: 85, Fat: 7g, Sodium: 1200mg, Carbs: 6g, Fiber: 2g, Sugar: 3g, Protein: 2g.

26. Lime Avocado and Cucumber Soup

Duration for preparing: 5 mins.
Ready in: 0 mins.
Persons: 4

Required Material:
- 2 avocados, pitted, peeled, and roughly cubed
- 2 cucumbers, sliced
- 950 ml vegetable stock
- 0.5g lemon zest, grated
- 15ml white vinegar
- 250 ml scallions
- A dash of salt, and some freshly powdered grains black pepper
- 15ml Oil of olive
- 15 gr cilantro

Instructions:
1. Puree the cucumbers, avocados, and the other components till creamy, then portion out the soup into separate servings and eat it for lunch.

Nutritional breakdown:

Calories: 190, Fat: 15g, Sodium: 960mg, Carbs: 14g, Fiber: 7g, Sugar: 4g, Protein: 4g.

27. Grilled Veggie Mix

Duration for preparing: 10 mins.
Ready in: 30 mins.
Persons: 4

Required Material:
- 450 gr cherry tomatoes, halved
- 2 eggplants, roughly cubed
- 475 gr radishes, halved
- 2 green bell peppers, halved, deseeded
- 5g chili powder
- 5g rosemary
- 60 ml balsamic vinegar
- A dash of salt, and some freshly powdered grains black pepper
- 30 ml Oil of olive
- 15g basil

Instructions:
1. Everything but the basil should be united in one plate and mixed together.
2. After spreading the veggies out on an already-prepared grill, you will need to cook them for 15 mins. on each side.
3. Divide the veggies among the dishes, then sprinkle each one with basil, and then serve.

Nutritional breakdown:

Calories: 194, Protein: 5 g, Fat: 10 g, Carbs: 24 g, Fiber: 10 g Sodium: 168 mg

28. Spinach and Cucumber Salad

Duration for preparing: 5 mins.
Ready in: 0 mins.
Persons: 4

Required Material:
- 450 gr cucumber, sliced
- 70 gr baby spinach
- 15g chili powder
- 30 ml Oil of olive
- 15 gr cilantro
- 30ml lemon juice
- A dash of salt, and some freshly powdered grains black pepper

Instructions:
1. Toss the cucumber, spinach, and the other elements of the salad together in a big container before serving.

Nutritional breakdown:

Calories: 85 Protein: 2 g Fat: 7 g, Carbs: 7 g, Fiber: 2 g Sodium: 157 mg

29. Curry Spinach Soup

Duration for preparing: 10 mins.
Ready in: 0 mins.
Persons: 4

Required Material:
- 235 ml almond milk
- 15g green curry paste
- 450 gr spinach leaves
- 15g cilantro
- A dash of salt, and some freshly powdered grains black pepper
- 950 ml veggie stock

Instructions:
1. Using a blender, incorporate the almond milk, curry paste, and all the other materials till they are perfectly smooth. Afterward, dish the soup in separate bowls for lunch.

Nutritional breakdown:
Calories: 82, Protein: 5 g, Fat: 3 g, Carbs: 12 g, Fiber: 5 g Sodium: 808 mg

30. Arugula and Artichokes Bowls

Duration for preparing: 5 mins.
Ready in: 0 mins.
Persons: 4

Required Material:
- 70 gr baby arugula
- 30 gr walnuts
- 225 gr canned artichoke hearts, drained and quartered
- 15ml balsamic vinegar
- 30g cilantro
- 30ml Oil of olive
- A dash of salt, and some freshly powdered grains black pepper
- 15ml lemon juice

Instructions:
1. Combine together the artichokes, arugula, walnuts, and additional ingredients. Mix well, and serve the meal as a side dish or a simple lunch.

Nutritional breakdown:
Calories: 120, Protein: 3g, Fat: 10 g, Carbs: 8 g, Fiber: 3 g Sodium: 358 mg

31. Keto Tofu and Spinach Casserole

Duration for preparing: 5 min
Ready in: 5 min
Serves: 4

Required Material:
- 1 block Firm Tofu, drained, pressed, and cut into cubes
- 1 Bell Pepper, diced
- ½ White Onion
- 30ml Oil of olive
- 100 grams Fresh Spinach
- 80g Diced Tomatoes
- 2g Paprika
- 2g Garlic Powder

Instructions:
1. Incorporate all ingredients in a pot.
2. Simmer for 5 mins.

Nutritional breakdown:
Calories: 158 Total Fat: 12g, Total Carbohydrates: 7g, Dietary Fiber: 3g, Sugars: 3g, Protein: 9g

32. Low-Carb Jambalaya

Duration for preparing: 10 min
Ready in: 10 min
Serves: 4

Required Material:
- 200 grams Seitan Sausages
- 400 grams Cauliflower, riced
- 240ml Vegetable Broth
- 1 Red Bell Pepper, diced
- 60g Frozen Peas
- Garlic, 3 cloves
- ½ White Onion, diced
- 45ml Oil of olive
- 5g Paprika
- 5g Oregano

Instructions:
1. Warm Oil of olive in a pan.
2. Add seitan and sear till slightly brown.
3. Add garlic, onions, and bell pepper. Sautee till aromatic.
4. Add cauliflower, broth, oregano, paprika, salt, and pepper.
5. Simmer for 6 mins
6. Eat hot.

Nutritional breakdown:

Calories: 205 Total Fat: 14g, Sodium: 423mg, Total Carbohydrates: 12g, Dietary Fiber: 5g, Sugars: 5g, Protein: 10g

33. Chili-Garlic Edamame

Duration for preparing: 5 min
Ready in: 10 min
Serves: 4

Required Material:
- 300 grams Edamame Pods
- 15ml Oil of Olive
- Garlic: 3 cloves
- 1.5g Chili Flakes, Red
- A dash of Salt

Instructions:
1. Steam edamame for 5 mins.
2. Warm Oil of olive in a pan.
3. Sautee garlic with chili till aromatic.
4. Include in steamed edamame and stir for a minute.
5. Season with salt.

Nutritional breakdown:

Calories: 101 Total Fat: 5g, Sodium: 77mg, Total Carbohydrates: 8g, Dietary Fiber: 4g, Sugars: 2g, Protein: 8g

34. Eggplant Pomodoro

Duration for preparing: 5 min
Ready in: 15 min
Serves: 4

Required Material:
- 1 Medium Eggplant, diced
- 240g Diced Tomatoes
- 60g Black Olives, sliced
- 4 cloves Garlic
- 30ml Wine Vinegar
- A dash of Pepper Flakes, red
- Salt & Pepper, as preferred
- 30ml Oil of olive
- 480g Shirataki Pasta
- Fresh Parsley

Instructions:
1. Oil of olive should be warmed in a pan.
2. Sautee garlic, red pepper flakes till aromatic.
3. Add eggplants, tomatoes, olives, and red wine vinegar. Stir till eggplants are soft.
4. Toss shirataki into the pan.
5. Season with spices.
6. Trim with parsley before distributing and eat.

Nutritional breakdown:

Calories: 117 Total Fat: 8g, Sodium: 492mg, Total Carbohydrates: 11g, Dietary Fiber: 6g, Sugars: 2g, Protein: 3g.

35. Vietnamese "Vermicelli" Salad

Duration for preparing: 5 min
Ready in: Serves: 4

Required Material:
- 100 grams Carrot, sliced into thin strips
- 200 grams Cucumbers, spiralized
- 30g Roasted Peanuts
- 60ml of each Fresh Mint and cilantro
- 5g Stevia
- 30ml Fresh Lime Juice
- 15ml Vegan Fish Sauce
- Garlic, 2 cloves
- A Green Chili
- 30ml Sesame Oil

Instructions:
1. Whisk together sugar, lime juice, sesame oil, fish sauce, garlic, and chopped chili.
2. Inside a bowl, toss together cucumbers, carrots, cucumbers, peanuts, mint, cilantro, and prepared dressing.
3. Serve chilled.

Nutritional breakdown:

Calories: 108, Fat: 7g, Carbohydrates: 10g, Fiber: 2g, Sugar: 5g, Protein: 3g

36. Homemade Vegan Sausages

Duration for preparing: 10 mins.
Ready in: 15 mins.
Serves: 4

Required Material:
- 120g Vital Wheat Gluten
- 30g Walnuts
- 30ml Onion
- 15ml Garlic
- 5g Cumin Powder
- 5g Smoked Paprika
- 2.5g Marjoram
- 1.25g each of: Salt, Oregano, Pepper
- 60ml Water
- 30ml Oil of olive

Instructions:
1. Include onions and garlic in a already warmed oiled pan and fry till soft.
2. Incorporate together onion, garlic and the rest of the components in a food processor. Blend into a homogenous texture.
3. Shape the mixture as desired.
4. Wrap each sausage in cling film, then with aluminum foil.
5. Steam for 30 mins..
6. Sausages may be later heated up in a pan, in the oven, or on the grill.

Nutritional breakdown:
Calories: 323, Protein: 33g, Fat: 15g, Carbohydrates: 12g, Fiber: 2g, Sugar: 2g, Sodium: 358mg.

37. Avocado, Endive and Asparagus Mix

Duration for preparing: 10 mins.
Ready in: 10 mins.
Persons: 4

Required Material:
- 2 avocados, peeled, pitted, and sliced
- 2 endives, shredded
- 4 asparagus spears, trimmed and halved
- 30ml sesame seeds
- 30ml avocado oil
- Juice of 1 lime
- A dash of Sea salt
- Black pepper
- 15g chives

Instructions:
1. Start by warming the oil in a pan, then include the endives, asparagus, avocados, and all the material.
2. Give everything a stir, then let it cook delicately for ten mins, either up slightly above the boiling point, before putting it on dishes and eating.

Nutritional breakdown:
Calories: 245, Protein: 4g, Fat: 22g, Carbohydrates: 13g, Fiber: 7g, Sodium: 60mg, Sugar: 2g

38. Collard Greens and Garlic Mix

Duration for preparing: 10 mins.
Ready in: 10 mins.
Persons: 4

Required Material:
- 30ml avocado oil
- 4 garlic cloves
- 4 bunches collard greens
- 1 tomato, cubed
- A dash of salt, and some freshly powdered grains black pepper
- Black pepper
- 7g almonds

Instructions:
1. Start by warming the oil that is already present in a skillet.
2. Include some crushed garlic in the mix, along with collard greens and the other ingredients.
3. Heat until the garlic is fragrant.
4. After thoroughly mixing all of the ingredients, continue cooking them for ten mins. at a low temperature, or just below the boiling point.
5. After that, portion the mixture out into bowls and serve.

Nutritional breakdown:
Calories: 121, Protein: 5g, Fat: 8g, Carbohydrates: 12g, Fiber: 6g, Sodium: 140mg, Sugar: 2g

39. Seitan Cauliflower Bowl

Duration for preparing: 10 mins.
Ready in: 22 mins. + 1 hour marinating
Persons: 4

Required Material:
- 60ml coconut aminos
- ½ lemon, juiced
- 15g garlic powder
- 15g swerve sugar
- 454g seitan, cut into strips
- 240ml Oil of olive
- 6 garlic cloves
- 600g cauliflower rice
- 30ml Oil of olive
- 4 large eggs
- 30g chopped fresh scallions, for garnishing

Instructions:
1. On a plate that is neither too large nor too little, mix the coconut, lemon juice, garlic granulate, and swerve sugar.
2. Make sure the seitan is well covered in the marinade after adding it, and then set it aside for an hour.
3. For 10 mins., or until browned and cooked through, sauté the seitan on both sides in hot sunflower oil in a wok that is neither too large nor too small. Prepare a serving tray for the seitan and set it aside.
4. About 30 seconds is all it takes for the garlic to start giving off its perfume in the pan. After around five mins. of stirring, during which time the cauliflower rice will have softened, season it with a mixture of table salt and black pepper. Put the food in the four bowls, divide it up evenly, and set them aside.
5. In the same wok, warm sunflower oil, after wiping it down with a paper towel.
6. Crack two eggs into the pan and fry them until they are golden, about a minute. Cook the remaining eggs in the leftover sunflower oil and serve one on top of the cauliflower rice in each dish.
7. Before serving, sprinkle some scallions on top and sprinkle the seitan over the whole dish.

Nutritional breakdown:

Calories: 518, Protein: 36g, Fat: 35g, Carbohydrates: 14g, Fiber: 4g, Sodium: 890mg, Sugar: 4g

40. Arugula Tomato Salad

Duration for preparing: 20 mins.
Persons: 2

Required Material:
- 60ml Oil of olive
- 240g cherry tomatoes, halved
- 90g arugula, washed, drained
- 1 small red onion
- 60g capers, canned, drained
- 30g basil, fresh

Instructions:
1. Add all ingredients into mixing bowl and toss.
2. Serve fresh and enjoy!

Nutritional breakdown:

Calories: 320, Protein: 4g, Fat: 31g, Carbohydrates: 10g, Fiber: 3g, Sodium: 684mg, Sugar: 4g

SOUPS AND STEWS

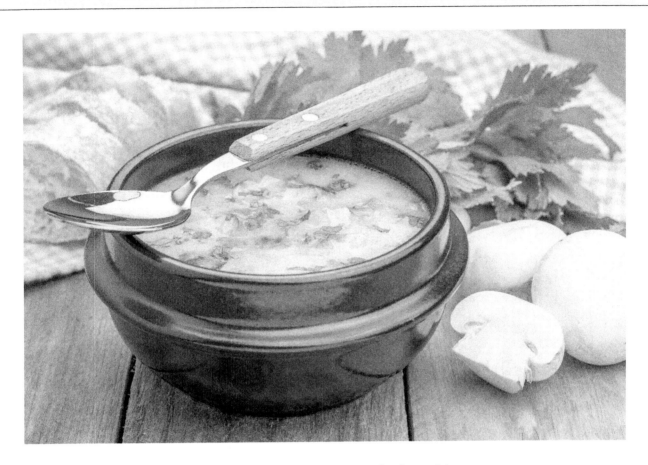

41. Beef Stew

Persons: 4
Duration for preparing: 10 mins.
Ready in: 2 hours

Required Material:
- 900 gr beef stew meat, cubed
- 1 red chili
- 1 brown onion
- 5 gr ghee, melted
- 30ml EVO oil
- One pinch of sea salt & black pepper
- 0.4g nutmeg, ground
- 1 garlic clove
- 113 gr white mushrooms, sliced
- 2g rosemary
- 5g fennel seeds
- 2 celery sticks
- 2 carrots, thinly sliced
- 1 lt beef stock
- 16 gr almond flour
- 1 sweet potato

Instructions:
1. After heating sunflower oil and the ghee together in a large pan include the shallot, chili, season to taste with spices, and continue cooking for another two to three mins..
2. After including the meat, give it a stir and let this boil for another five mins.
3. After tossing in the mushrooms, garlic, stock, fennel, rosemary, and nutmeg, bring the ingredients to a boil, cover, and then cook for 1 hour and 10 mins..
4. After incorporating the potato, celery, and carrots, stir everything together, cover the

pot, and let it till are soft.
5. After thoroughly mixing the flour with one cup of the stew's liquid in a basin, pour the mixture over the stew and continue the cook for fifteen mins.
6. Enjoy!

Nutritional breakdown:

Calories: 582, Total fat: 34g, Saturated fat: 11g, Cholesterol: 139mg, Sodium: 832mg, Carbs: 25g, Fiber: 6g, Sugars: 8g, Protein: 44g

42. Turkey Soup

Persons: 6
Duration for preparing: 15 mins.
Ready in: 40 mins.

Required Material:

- 1 yellow onion
- 1 tablespoon (15 gr) avocado oil
- 3 thyme springs
- 3 garlic cloves, finely
- 700 gr fresh tomatoes, peeled
- 170 gr tomato paste
- 60 ml of water
- 454 gr turkey meat, ground, fried
- 400 gr of beef stock
- 6 mushrooms
- 1 small red bell pepper
- 60 gr black olives

Instructions:

1. Put the oil in a pan and warm it, then add half of the shallot, garlic, and thyme. Blend ingredients together, continue cooking for another 5 mins..
2. Tomatoes, concentrated tomatoes, and water should be included in a pot and thoroughly mixed before bringing it to a boil. The mixture should then be allowed to simmer for twenty mins. at a temperature that is neither extremely high nor extremely low.
3. A blender should be used to thoroughly combine these ingredients.
4. Include the turkey, give it a stir, and continue cooking it for another four mins. while breaking it up with a fork after heating a saucepan.
5. Now incorporate the blended soup and the beef stock, stir well and continue cooking gently for an additional five mins. with the remaining shallot, mushrooms, and bell pepper.
6. Distribute olives around the top of each dish before filling with soup and serving!

Nutritional breakdown:

Calories: 236, Total fat: 12g, Saturated fat: 2g, Cholesterol: 67mg, Sodium: 562mg, Carbs: 15g, Fiber: 4g, Sugars: 8g, Protein: 19g

43. Tomato and Basil Soup

Persons: 4
Duration for preparing: 10 mins.
Ready in: 35 mins.

Required Material:

- 1,5 kg fresh tomatoes, peeled, crushed
- 473 ml tomato juice
- 473 ml chicken stock
- 113 gr coconut butter, melted
- 14 basil leaves, torn
- 240 ml coconut milk
- A dash of salt, and some freshly powdered grains black pepper

Instructions:

1. Unite the chopped tomatoes, tomato juice, and the stock. Boil over a heat that is neither very high nor extremely low for an extended period of time. Let thirty mins. at a temperature either just below the boiling point.
2. After adding the basil leaves one at a time, pour the mixture into a blender and give it a good spin before transferring it back to the saucepan.
3. Bring the soup back up to temperature, then incorporate the butter, salt, pepper, and coconut milk before whisking. After continuing to simmer the soup over low heat for a further four mins. the soup should then be served in individual bowls and enjoy it!

Nutritional breakdown:

Calories: 392, Total fat: 33g, Saturated fat: 25g, Sodium: 653mg, Carbs: 21g, Fiber: 5g, Sugars: 13g, Protein: 7g

44. Chicken and Mushroom Soup

Persons: 4
Duration for preparing: 15 mins.
Ready in: 60 mins.

Required Material:
- 10ml coconut oil, melted
- 3 carrots
- 1 yellow onion
- 1 zucchini
- 425 gr mushrooms
- 460 gr chicken meat, already cooked and shredded
- 4g rosemary
- 1 teaspoon thyme
- 15 ml apple cider vinegar
- 1 teaspoon cumin, ground
- 590 gr chicken stock
- A dash of salt, and some freshly powdered grains black pepper

Instructions:
1. After warming oil that has been added in a skillet, insert the carrots and shallot, toss and continue frying gently for 5 mins..
2. After amalgamating, continue cooking for another ten mins. with the zucchini and mushrooms in the same pan.
3. After introducing the chicken meat, rosemary, thyme, Apple Cider, and cumin and stirring the mixture, bring all of the ingredients together to a boil, then reduce the heat to a level that is neither very high nor very low and let it cook slowly for forty mins..
4. After flavoring the concoction with salt and pepper, give it one more turn, and then put it into bowls so that it may be enjoyed!

Nutritional breakdown:
Calories: 383 kcal, Total fat: 14 g, Cholesterol: 144 mg, Sodium: 422 mg, Carbs: 18 g, Fiber: 4 g, Sugars: 8 g, Protein: 46 g

45. Coconut Chicken Soup

Persons: 6
Duration for preparing: 15 mins.
Ready in: 30 mins.

Required Material:
- 2 stalks of celery
- 120ml coconut oil melted
- 2 carrots
- 60 g of arrow starch
- 1.4 liters of chicken broth
- 2g dried parsley
- 120ml of water
- 1 bay leaf
- A pinch of salt and black pepper
- 1g dried thyme
- 360 ml of coconut milk
- 450 g of organic chicken meat, already cooked and cut into cubes

Instructions:
1. In a large saucepan that already has oil that has been warmed to a temperature that is neither very high nor extremely low, carrots and celery are then added. After this, the mixture is given a stir, and it is let to simmer for 10 mins.. After the stock has been added, you should give the mixture a toss before bringing it to a boil.
2. Using the dish, combine the arrowroot powder with a half cup of water. After giving the mixture a thorough stirring, transfer it to the pot.
3. After adding the parsley, sea salt, pepper, bay leaf, and thyme, toss and then let it stew gently for fifteen mins..
4. After adding the meat and amalgamating to the coconut milk, continue cooking the dish over low heat for one more minute and then serve it in bowls. Enjoy!

Nutritional breakdown:
Calories: 377 kcal, Fat: 30g, Saturated Fat: 21g, Cholesterol: 51mg, Carbs: 13g, Fiber: 2g, Sugar: 3g, Protein: 16g, Sodium: 751mg

46. Lemon Soup

Persons: 4
Duration for preparing: 10 mins.
Ready in: 10 mins.

Required Material:
- 1,4 lt shellfish stock

- 1 garlic
- 15 ml coconut oil, melted
- 2 eggs
- 120 ml lemon juice
- A dash of salt, and some freshly powdered grains black pepper
- 8 gr arrowroot powder
- 5g cilantro

Instructions:
1. Put to warm the oil that is already there in a saucepan over a heat source that is neither very high nor extremely low. Add garlic, then let it fry steadily for two mins..
2. After the addition of the stock, give the mixture a swirl, then lower the heat to a low setting to continue cooking the mixture gently.
3. Once fully incorporated eggs, salt, pepper, lemon juice, and arrowroot together inside the saucepan, continue cooking for an additional four mins..
4. When you are done, divide the mixture amongst many bowls, and then sprinkle each one with the cilantro into very thin bits!

Nutritional breakdown:
Calories: 156, Fat: 9g, Cholesterol: 116mg, Sodium: 231mg, Carbs: 9g, Fiber: 1g, Sugars: 2g, Protein: 10g

47. Black Bean Soup

Duration for preparing: 10 mins.
Ready in: 15 mins.
Persons: 4

Required Material:
- 30ml Oil of olive
- 1 of each onion green bell pepper,carrot
- 4 garlic cloves
- 2 can of 400 gr black beans, drained and rinsed
- 475 ml vegetable stock
- 0.5g ground cumin
- 5g sea salt
- 4 gr chopped cilantro, for garnish

Instructions:
1. To make the sunflower oil shimmer in a large soup pot, warm it for as long as it reaches that temperature.
2. Continue cooking after including bell pepper, onion, and carrot till the vegetables are soft. Wait for the garlic to become fragrant, which should take around 30 seconds. At this time, add the black beans, vegetable stock, cumin, and salt. Cook the mixture turning it often, over neither very high nor very low heat (10 mins).
3. Get rid of the food from the heat. After softly mashing the bean, leave some bean pieces in the soup. A smoother final product will come by working the soup in a blender or food processor.
4. To serve, reach the point of a boil and top with thinly cut cilantro.

Nutritional breakdown:
Calories: 283, Fat: 8g, Sodium: 682mg, Carbs: 43g, Fiber: 15g, Sugars: 5g, Protein: 12g

48. Creamy Garlic-Spinach Rotini Soup

Duration for preparing: 10 mins.
Ready in: 15 mins.
Persons: 4

Required Material:
- 5ml Oil of olive
- 150 gr chopped mushrooms
- 0.5g plus a pinch of salt
- 4 garlic cloves
- 2 peeled carrots or ½ red bell pepper
- 1,4 lt Economical Vegetable Broth or water
- Pinch freshly ground black pepper
- 100 gr rotini or gnocchi
- 180 ml unsweetened nondairy milk
- 30 gr nutritional yeast
- 200 gr chopped fresh spinach
- 30 gr pitted black olives or sun-dried tomatoes
- Herbed Croutons for topping (optional)

Instructions:
1. For heating the sunflower oil, place it in a heavy-duty soup pot and set the flame to medium.
2. Add some salt and mushrooms to the food. The mushrooms should be stir-fried for

about four minutes till they are as tender as you want them.
3. Keep sautéing for another minute after you add the carrots and fresh garlic (if using). Include salt, black pepper and garlic powder (if using), plus vegetables on your list.
4. Bring it to a boil and immediately add the pasta. Ten minutes should be enough time to get the pasta to the perfect al dente texture.
5. Take away the pan from the heat and, while stirring constantly, add the milk, nutritional yeast, spinach, and olives. If you want, you may sprinkle some croutons on top.
6. The food may be kept in an airtight container in the fridge for up to a week, or in the freezer for up to a month.

Nutritional breakdown:
Calories: 250, Protein: 14g, Total fat: 5g, Carbs: 38g; Fiber: 6g

49. White And Wild Mushroom Barley Soup

Duration for preparing: 5 mins.
Ready in: 50 mins.
Persons: 4 to 6

Required Material:
- 15ml Oil of olive
- A onion
- One carrot
- Two celery ribs
- 340 gr white mushrooms
- 225 gr cremini, shiitake
- 200 gr pearl barley
- 1,65 lt mushroom broth
- 2g dried dillweed
- A dash of salt, and some freshly powdered grains black pepper
- 30g fresh parsley

Instructions:
1. Shallots, carrots, and celery may be added after being thinly sliced in an oiled stockpot already warmed. Ten minutes, covered, should be enough time to get them soft.
2. Take the lid off and stir in the dill, mushrooms, barley, and broth as long as everything is evenly distributed. Add spices to taste.
3. Bring to a boil, uncovered, and cook for about 40 minutes, barley and vegetables must be tender.
4. Before serving, give it a taste after adding the parsley and adjust the seasoning as needed.

Nutritional breakdown: for portion:
Calories: 214, Fat: 4.6 g, Carbs: 38.7 g, Protein: 7.2g, Fibers: 9.4g

50. Italian Wedding Soup

Duration for preparing: 10 mins.
Ready in: 15 mins.
Persons: 4

Required Material:
- 5 ml Oil of olive
- 2 carrots, peeled and chopped
- ½ onion
- 3 or 4 garlic cloves, or 2.5g garlic powder
- Salt
- 2 lt water or Economical Vegetable Broth
- 200 gr orzo or pearl couscous
- 5 gr dried herbs
- Freshly ground black pepper
- 1 recipe of quinoa meatballs
- 100 gr chopped greens, such as spinach, kale, or chard

Instructions:
1. Olive oil should be warmed in a big stockpot that has been prepared on moderately high heat.
2. The carrots, onion, and garlic (if using fresh) should be added, along with a little bit of salt. Fry for 3 to 4 minutes., as long as softened. Orzo, water, and dried herbs should be included, along with garlic powder (if it is being used). The soup should be seasoned according to preference before arriving at a boil.
3. Simmer the orzo for approximately ten minutes, to reach the desired consistency. After adding the meatballs and greens, mix everything together, till the greens have become wilted.
4. Experiment with flavor, and add more spices

as desired.

Nutritional breakdown:
Calories: 287; Protein: 14g; Total fat: 5g; Saturated fat: 1g; Carbs: 49g; Fiber: 7g

51. Spinach and Watermelon Soup

Persons: 3
Duration for preparing: 10 mins.
Ready in: 0

Required Material:
- One avocado
- 2 bunches spinach
- 360g watermelon
- A single bunch cilantro
- 2 lemons, only juice plus
- A cucumber
- 120ml amino of coconut

Instructions:
1. Put all of the ingredients that are needed into the container of your blender and give them a good whirl, then split them into individual dishes and enjoy.

Nutritional breakdown:
Calories: 431, Protein: 13g, Fat: 28g, Carbohydrates: 46g, Fiber: 17g, Sugar: 22g, Sodium: 1264mg

52. Broccoli Soup

Duration for preparing: 10 mins.
Ready in: 20 mins.
Persons: 4

Required Material:
- 1 yellow onion
- 30ml Oil of olive
- 1 celery stick
- Zest of ½ lemon, grated
- 1-quart veggie stock
- 500ml water
- 2g cumin, ground
- 1 broccoli head, florets separated
- 3 garlic cloves
- 2 bay leaves
- Juice of ½ lemon
- A dash of salt, and some freshly powdered grains black pepper

For the pesto:
- 60g almonds
- 1 garlic clove
- 30ml lemon juice
- 30ml Oil of olive
- 60g green olives

Instructions:
1. Stir in the onion, lemon zest, and a little salt into the 30 ml of olive oil that has been heated in a big pot; fry for 3 minutes.
2. Stir in the celery and three garlic cloves, and continue cooking for a further minute.
3. Stir in the stock, cumin, water, and blackpepper; cover, carry to a boil, and continue to cook for ten mins.
4. Stir in the bay leaves and broccoli, then return the lid and simmer for a further 6 minutes.
5. Take away soup from flame, and place inside a blender after discarding bay leaves,
6. Pulse once more, add the juice of half a lemon, then transfer everything back into the saucepan and reheat.
7. In the meantime, puree almonds, garlic clove, lemon juice, olive oil, and green olives as long as a smooth paste forms.
8. Put the soup in the dishes and sprinkle each serving with the freshly prepared pesto.
9. Enjoy!

Nutritional breakdown:
Calories: 373, Protein: 12g, Fat: 29g, Carbohydrates: 21g, Fiber: 8g, Sugar: 7g, Sodium: 1028mg

53. Hot & Sour Tofu Soup

Duration for preparing: 40 Mins.
Ready in: 15 Mins.
Persons:3

Required Material:
- 170 to 198g firm or extra-firm tofu
- 5ml Oil of olive
- 150g sliced mushrooms
- 100g finely chopped cabbage
- 1 garlic clove
- ½-inch piece fresh gingerd

- Salt
- 950ml or Economical Vegetable Broth
- 30ml rice vinegar or apple cider vinegar
- 30ml soy sauce
- 5ml toasted sesame oil
- 5g sugar
- Pinch red pepper flakes
- A white and light green parts of scallion

Instructions:
1. Press your tofu before you start: Put it between several layers of paper towels and place a heavy pan or book (with a waterproof cover or protected with plastic wrap) on top. Leave for 30 minutes. Throw away the used paper towels. Cubed the tofu to a half-inch in size.
2. Olive oil should be warmed in a big soup pot.
3. Put in the cabbage, garlic, ginger, and a bit of salt along with the mushrooms. The veggies should be sautéed for 7–8 minutes.
4. Include the sugar, red pepper flakes, red wine vinegar, soy sauce, sesame oil, water, and tofu.
5. Get it boiling for around 10 mins.
6. Spread the scallion on top before serving.
7. A week in the fridge or a month in the freezer is all the time you need to store leftovers in an airtight container.

Nutritional breakdown:
Calories: 124, Protein: 10g, Fat: 6g, Carbohydrates: 10g, Fiber: 2g, Sugar: 6g, Sodium: 1344mg

54. Autumn Medley Stew

Duration for preparing: 5 Mins.
Ready in: 60 Mins.
Persons: 4 To 6

Required Material:
- 30ml Oil of olive
- 226.8g seitan, homemade
- 1 large yellow onion
- 2 garlic
- One piece of each vegetable: large russet potato, carrot, parsnip, butternut squash, head savoy cabbage
- (411g) A can tomatoes
- 225g chickpeas, drained and rinsed
- 480ml vegetable broth,
- 120ml dry white wine
- 0.5g dried marjoram
- 0.5g dried thyme
- 40g angel hair pasta (crumbled)

Instructions:
1. Prepare and warm one-half of the oil till shimmering in a big pan. After adding the seitan, fry it for five more minutes to brown both sides. Flavor with salt and pepper.
2. Warm the remaining part of the oil in a big pan over a low-to-medium heat source. Include garlic and shallot. Tenderize vegetables by cooking for 5 minutes. Butternut squash, potatoes, carrots, and parsnips should be cooked together. Cover and keep on the flame for 10 minutes till the vegetables are soft.
3. Once adding salt, pepper, marjoram, thyme, broth, wine, tomatoes, and chickpeas, mix them. Cook the veggies with the lid on for 45 mins, tossing occasionally.
4. Now incorporate the seitan and noodles, boil for about ten mins as long as the pasta is al dente and the flavors have blended. Serve meals hot or warm.

Nutritional breakdown:
Calories: 384, Total Fat: 11.9g, Saturated Fat: 1.7g, Sodium: 891mg, Total Carbohydrates: 46.6g, Dietary Fiber: 12.1g, Sugar: 9.1g, Protein: 20.9g

55. Tuscan White Bean Soup

Duration for preparing: 10 Mins.
Ready in: 15 Mins.
Persons: 4

Required Material:
- 5ml to 10ml Oil of olive
- 1 onion
- 4 garlic cloves, or 1 teaspoon garlic powder
- 2 carrots, peeled and chopped
- Salt
- 14.8g dried herbs
- A dash of black pepper and flakes of red

pepper
- 946ml Economical Vegetable Broth or water
- 425g white beans (cannellini, navy, or great Northern)
- 30ml freshly squeezed lemon juice
- 120g chooped greens (kale, spinach, arugula, chard)

Instructions:
1. Preparing the Ingredients.
2. Olive oil should be heated in a big stockpot before including the carrots, onion, and garlic (if using fresh), and season with a little bit of salt.
3. Prepare the vegetables for about five minutes, stirring them a few times, until they acquire a light brown color. After inserting the dry herbs, as well as the garlic powder, black pepper, and red pepper flakes, toss everything together so that everything is well distributed.
4. To finish heating the soup, unite the bean puree, the other salt, and the vegetable broth. If you want the broth to be a little bit creamier, you can purée one to two cups of the soup in a countertop blender and then return it to the saucepan after puréeing it. Alternatively, you may use a hand blender to purée roughly a quarter of the beans that are already in the saucepan.
5. It is time to include the lemon juice and the greens and let some time for the greens to wilt before serving the soup.
6. The leftovers can be stored in the refrigerator for up to one week or in the freezer for up to one month if they are placed in an airtight container.

Nutritional breakdown:
Calories: 266 Total Fat: 4.6g, Sodium: 956mg, Potassium: 758mg, Total Carbohydrates: 45g, Dietary Fiber: 13g, Sugars: 5g, Protein: 14g

56. Mexican Fideo Soup with Pinto Beans

Duration for preparing: 5 Mins.
Ready in: 25 Mins.
Persons: 4

Required Material:
- 44ml Oil of olive
- 1 medium onion
- 3 garlic cloves
- 226g fideo, vermicelli, or angel hair pasta
- 1 (411g) can tomatoes
- 356g cooked or 1 (439g) can pinto beans, rinsed
- (113g) 1 can green chiles
- 2.6g cumin
- 0.5g oregano
- 1.4lt vegetable broth, homemade
- 20g cilantro

Instructions:
1. A Half amount of the oil should be heated in a big soup pot. Put a lid on the pan after including the onion for approximately 10 minutes. Now add the garlic. A slotted spoon may be used to remove the onion mixture.
2. Noodles should be cooked in the same pot with the remaining part of the oil and which should take around 5 to 7 minutes. Take care that the noodles do not become burned.
3. Mix in the broth, salt and pepper to taste, and the tomatoes, beans, chiles, cumin, and oregano. Add the onion combination and cook, stirring occasionally, for 10 to 15 minutes, or until the veggies and noodles are cooked. Serve in bowls topped with chopped cilantro

Nutritional breakdown:
Calories: 409, Fat: 16g, Carbohydrates: 55g, Fiber: 10g, Sugar: 6g, Protein: 14g, Sodium: 1318mg

57. Lamb and Coconut Stew

Persons: 4
Duration for preparing: 15 mins.
Ready in: 1 hour and 50 mins.

Required Material:
- 680g lamb meat, cubed
- 15ml coconut oil, melted
- ½ red chili, seedless and chopped
- 1 brown onion
- 3 garlic cloves
- 2 celery sticks

- 12g garam masala powder
- 5g fennel seeds
- A dash of salt, and some freshly powdered grains black pepper
- 6g turmeric powder
- 7g ghee, melted
- 400ml coconut milk
- 240ml water
- 15ml lemon juice
- 2 carrots
- A handful parsley leaves, finely chopped

Instructions:
1. Brown the lamb for 4 minutes on each side with oil in a pan.
2. Stir in the celery, chili, and onion. Cook for 1 minute with the heat turned down to medium and the garam masala, garlic, ghee, fennel, and turmeric added while stirring.
3. Flavor with salt and pepper, then incorporate in tomato paste, coconut milk, and water. Boil, cover, and let on the slow flame for an hour.
4. Toss occasionally for a further 40 minutes after adding the carrots.
5. Include some freshly squeezed lemon juice and chopped parsley before serving. Enjoy!

Nutritional breakdown:
Calories: 579, Protein: 37 g, Fat: 45 g, Carbohydrates: 10 g, Fiber: 3 g, Sodium: 296 mg

58. Veggie and Kale Stew

Persons: 6
Duration for preparing: 10 mins.
Ready in: 1 hour and 10 mins.

Required Material:
- 1.8kg mixed root vegetables (parsnips, carrots, rutabagas, beets, celery root, turnips
- 90ml EVO oil
- 1 garlic head, cloves
- 120ml yellow onion
- Black pepper to taste
- 740ml fresh tomatoes, peeled
- 15g tomato paste
- 480g kale leaves, torn
- 5g oregano

Instructions:
1. In a baking dish, mix all root vegetables with black pepper, half of the oil, and garlic, toss to coat.
2. Bake (230°C - 45 mins).
3. Introduce onions in a pan with already warmed oil, and sauté (3 mins).
4. Include tomato paste, tomatoes, spices, veggies, kale and the oregano, and leave on the flame for 5 more mins.
5. Dish up into separate bowls, and eat!!

Nutritional breakdown:
Calories: 305, Protein: 6 g, Fat: 18 g, Carbohydrates: 34 g, Fiber: 9 g, Sodium: 123 mg

59. Lemony Lentil and Rice Soup

Duration for preparing: 15 mins.
Ready in: 1hour 10 mins.
Persons: 6

Required Material:
- 30ml Oil of olive
- 1 of: onion, carrot, celery rib
- 295ml brown lentils
- 180ml brown rice
- (411g) A can tomatoes
- 480ml tomato sauce
- Two bay leaves
- 1g cumin
- 1.14lt water
- Black-pepper
- 15ml lemon, only juice
- 30g parsley
- Salt

Instructions:
1. Warm the oil in a big stockpot. Include the chopped onion, carrot, and celery in the dish. Cook under cover for about ten minutes till tender.
2. The lentils, rice, tomatoes, tomato juice, bay leaves, cumin, water, salt, and pepper should all be added at this point. Raise to a boil and continue to simmer, uncovered, for about 60 mins.
3. At the time of serving, take out the bay leaves then add the parsley and lemon juice

and whisk everything together. After tasting, make any required adjustments to the seasoning, and then serve.

Nutritional breakdown:
Calories: 327, Total Fat: 6.5 g, Sodium: 563 mg, Total Carbohydrates: 52 g, Dietary Fiber: 14, Sugars: 7 g, Protein: 16 g

60. Roasted Vegetable Bisque

Duration for preparing: 10 mins.
Ready in: 15 mins.
Persons: 6

Required Material:
- A large onion
- 2 medium carrots
- One large russet potato
- A medium zucchini
- One large ripe tomato
- 2 garlic
- 30ml olive-oil
- 5g savory and thyme
- Salt & pepper
- 960ml broth (vegetable)
- 15g parsley

Instructions:
1. Start your oven temperature up to 200 degrees C. Put vegetables in a tin that has been lightly greased. Spray with oil and flavor with salt, pepper, and herbs of choice. Cover with foil securely and bake for 30 minutes, or as long as tender. Eliminate the foil and cook for a further 30 minutes after stirring once, till the veggies are gently browned.
2. The broth is boiled in a big soup pot, before adding the veggies. Keep on flame for 15 minutes.
3. If necessary, work in batches and puree the soup before returning it to the saucepan. Try it out, and if the seasonings are not sufficient, flavor again.
4. Serve by ladling into dishes and topping with parsley.

Nutritional breakdown:
Calories: 152, Total Fat: 5.5 g, Cholesterol: 0 mg, Sodium: 658 mg, Total Carbohydrates: 24 g, Dietary Fiber: 4 g, Sugars: 5 g, Protein: 4 g

SALADS RECIPES

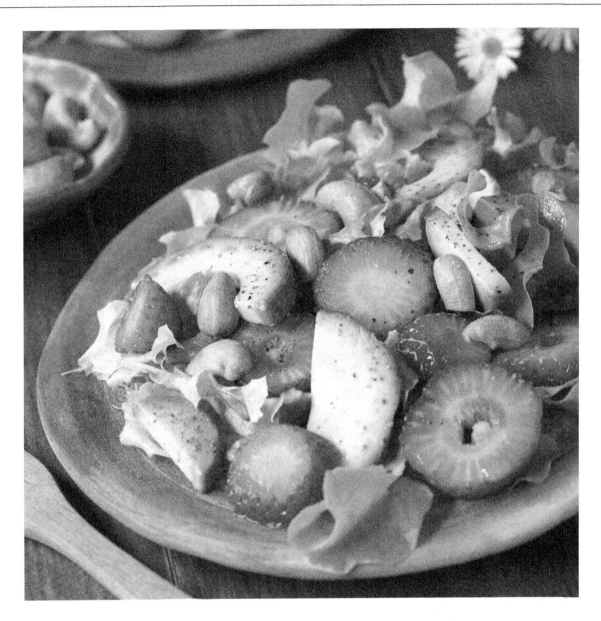

61. Mango salad

Duration for preparing: 5 mins
Persons: 2

Required Material:
- 10 gr seeded and jalapeño pepper
- 30 gr chopped fresh cilantro
- Juice of 1 lime
- 3 pitted and cubed ripe mangos
- 5 gr red onion

Instructions:
1. Mix everything you need in a salad bowl. Toss the salad well.

Nutritional breakdown:
Calories: 331, Fat:5 g, Carbs:28.1 g, Protein:1 g, Sugars:27 g, Sodium:3.4 mg

62. Shrimp and Asparagus Salad

Duration for preparing: 10 mins
Persons: 4

Required Material:
- 2 halved cherry tomatoes
- Cracked black pepper
- 340 gr trimmed fresh asparagus spears
- 454 gr frozen peeled and cooked shrimp
- Cracker bread
- 120 gr watercress
- 120 ml bottled light raspberry

Instructions:
1. Prepare the asparagus in a small amount of hot, lightly salted water for three minutes in a large, flat dish that has been covered. A sieve is used to drain the asparagus. Pass through a stream of cold water to cool down fast.
2. Put some asparagus on each of dinner plates, then add some lettuce, prawns and cherry tomatoes on top. Pour the dressing over the top.
3. Cracked black pepper should be put on top, and sandwich bread should be served on the side.

Nutritional breakdown:
Calories: 155.5, Fat:1.4 g, Carbs:15 g, Protein:22 g, Sugars:1 g, Sodium:324 mg

63. Carrot and walnut salad

Duration for preparing: 10 mins
Persons: 2

Required Material:
- 30 gr chopped walnuts
- 1 peeled, cored, and sliced apple
- Parsley leaves
- 1 peeled and grated carrot
- 21 gr honey

Instructions:
1. It is recommended that honey be drizzled over the shredded carrots.
2. Make a salad by arranging the carrots, apples, and walnuts on the serving dish in alternating layers.
3. For a decorative touch, sprinkle over some chopped parsley leaves.

Nutritional breakdown:
Calories: 206, Fat: 11g, Carbs: 28g, Protein: 3g, Sugars: 21g, Sodium: 13mg

64. Pickled onion salad

Duration for preparing: 1 hour
Persons: 4

Required Material:
- 4 chopped spring onions
- 15 gr chopped fresh cilantro
- 25 gr brown sugar
- 15 ml lime juice
- 120 ml cider vinegar
- 2 thinly sliced red onions
- 4 lettuce leaves
- 10 ml Oil of olive

Instructions:
1. Using a salad bowl, mix the onion with the Cider Vinegar, oil, and sugar.
2. Keep covered and chill in the fridge for 1 hour.
3. Include some fresh lime juice and cilantro.
4. Position on a bed of lettuce leaves.

Nutritional breakdown:
Calories: 68, Fat: 2g, Carbs: 12g, Protein: 1g, Sugars: 9g, Sodium: 3mg

65. Strawberries and Avocado Salad

Duration for preparing: 5 mins
Persons: 2

Required Material:
- 300 gr halved strawberries
- 2 pitted and peeled avocados
- 10 gr chopped mint
- 1 peeled and sliced banana

Instructions:
1. The recipe should begin by having the bananas, strawberries, mint, and avocados mixed together. After that, the combination should be tossed and then served at room temperature.

2. Dish up!

Nutritional breakdown:
Calories: 312, Fat: 22 g, Carbs: 31g, Protein: 4g, Sugars: 17g, Sodium: 11mg

66. Pickled Grape Salad with Pear, Taleggio, and Walnuts

Duration for preparing: 15 mins
Persons: 3

Required Material:
- 200g sliced taleggio cheese
- 60 ml red wine vinegar
- 25 g light brown sugar
- 2 handfuls fresh watercress
- 100g halved red grapes
- 1 wedged pear
- 50g halved walnut

Instructions:
1. Toast the walnut halves in a cast-iron pan or pot with a level base over low to medium heat until they become brown and smell nutty. Leave to cool.
2. Mix the light brown sugar and red wine Apple Cider in a plate and allow sit for five minutes to dissolve.
3. Add grapes to the sweet and sour mixture and toss. After 10 minutes, continue with the recipe.
4. Distribute the watercress among three plates or all of the servings on a large platter, then evenly put the pear pieces and taleggio cheese on top.
5. Reuse the marinade after removing the grapes.
6. Whisk sunflower oil into the pickling marinade.
7. Place the pickled grapes in a random pattern over the salad, then sprinkle 3–4 teaspoons of the dressing beyond the pale.
8. Finally, sprinkle the walnut halves with toasted walnuts and enjoy immediately.

Nutritional breakdown:
Calories: 440, Fat: 32,3 g, Carbs: 19,7 g, Protein:19,3 g, Sugars: 15,7 g, Sodium:547 mg

67. Fresh Fruit Salad

Duration for preparing: 15 mins
Persons: 3

Required Material:
- 1 halved and sliced ripe banana
- 170 g sliced and halved strawberries,
- 170 g julienned granny smith apples
- 1 g salt
- 340 g chopped ripe pineapple
- 170 g sliced and quartered kiwi
- 340 g chopped ripe mango

Instructions:
1. First cut the bananas so they are about a centimeter thick, and then cut them in half lengthwise.
2. Cut the mangoes and kiwis up into small pieces to get the most flavour out of them.
3. Once you are done chopping all the fruit, put it in the dish and apply some salt on top.
4. Give it a good stir to mix everything together, and enjoy!

Nutritional breakdown:
Calories: 319, Fat: 2 g, Carb: 81 g, Protein: 4g

68. Dried apricot sauce

Duration for preparing: 2 hours
Persons: 4

Required Material:
- 100 g sugar
- 113-gram dried apricots
- 35 gr cornstarch

Instructions:
1. Put the apricots that have been dried into a dish, and then pour boiling water over them until they are fully covered. Allow them to soak for anywhere between one and two hours.
2. After bringing the water in which the dried apricots are suspended to a boil, continue the cooking process for the subsequent thirty minutes.
3. Following the addition of sugar, the liquid is brought back up to a boil while being stirred consistently during the process.

4. In order to prepare the cornflour solution, combine cornflour and water in a 1:4 ratio, then whisk the mixture until it is smooth.
5. While the dehydrated apricot sauce is already simmering, add the cornflour solution to the pot. After five minutes, give it a stir and then remove it from the heat immediately thereafter.
6. Serve as a garnish for any of your go-to sweets by spreading it on top.

Nutritional breakdown:
Calories: 155, Fat:0.1 g, Carbs: 40,2 g, Protein:0.6g, Sugars: 34,1 g, Sodium: 1mg

69. Tomato, Cucumber, and Basil Salad

Duration for preparing: 10 mins
Serving: 4

Required Material:
- 1 garlic clove
- 0,5 gr freshly ground black pepper
- 15 ml Oil of olive
- 1 thinly sliced small onion
- 2 medium cucumbers
- 4 quartered ripe medium tomatoes
- 10 gr chopped fresh basil
- 45 ml red wine vinegar

Instructions:
1. To remove the seeds from the cucumbers, first, peel them, then split them in half, and last use a spoon to scrape them out.
2. The cucumber should be halved lengthwise, and then each half should be placed in its own dish. Onion, tomatoes, and basil leaves should all be combined at this point. Place any leftover ingredients in a separate bowl and give them a thorough stirring to ensure that everything is combined.
3. After pouring the dressing over the salad, tossing it will ensure that it is distributed equally throughout the salad's components. You have the option of serving it right away, or you can cover it, put it in the refrigerator, and wait to serve it until you are ready.

Nutritional breakdown:
Calories: 80, Fat: 5g, Carbs: 9g, Protein: 2g, Sugars: 5g, Sodium: 10mg

70. Caramelized Onion and Beet Salad

Duration for preparing: 10 mins.
Ready in: 40 mins.
Persons: 4

Required Material:
- 3 medium golden beets
- 240 gr sliced sweet or Vidalia onions
- 1 teaspoon extra-virgin Oil or no-beef broth
- Pinch baking soda
- A pinch of salt, to taste
- 30 ml rice vinegar, white wine vinegar, or balsamic vinegar

Instructions:
1. Clean the beets after chopping the greens.
2. water to a big saucepan with a steamer basket inside.
3. After adding the beets, boil, coat, and steam for 35 mins, or till a knife can easily be put into the center.
4. In a dry skillet, fry the onions for five minutes, stirring constantly.
5. After adding the sunflower oil and bicarbonate of soda, simmer steadily for 5 minutes just below or slightly over the boiling point, stirring often. Stir the salt and season to taste before removing the pan from the heat. Set aside the mixture in a big bowl.
6. After cooking, rinse and chill the beets. Rub beets with a paper towel to quickly remove their skins. Before adding the shallots, chop the potatoes into wedges. Drizzle vinegar over everything and stir.
7. Distribute the beets among four wide-mouthed jars. Put the lids on once they cool.

Nutritional breakdown:
Calories: 109, Fat: 2,5g, Protein: 3g, Carbs: 20g, Fiber: 4g, Sugar: 13g, Sodium: 225mg

71. Spinach Salad With Orange-Dijon Dressing

Duration for preparing: 10 mins.
Ready in: 0 mins.
Persons: 4

Required Material:
- 30g Dijon mustard
- 30ml Oil of olive
- 60ml fresh orange juice
- 5g agave nectar
- 2.5g salt
- 0.5g black pepper
- 30g parsley
- 15g green onions
- 200g fbaby spinach
- A navel orange
- Half small onion

Instructions:
1. Make sure that the brown mustard, oil, orange juice, agave nectar, salt, pepper, parsley, and green onion are well blended by pulsing them in a food processor or blending them in a blender.
2. Combine everything very well, then set it aside.
3. In a large bowl, combine the orange and shallot with the shallot and spinach. The meal is now ready to be served, after adding the dressing and giving everything a quick stir.

Nutritional breakdown:
Calories: 102, Fat: 7.6g, Sodium: 383mg, Carbohydrates: 8.7g, Fiber: 2.1g, Sugars: 5.1g, Protein: 1.8g

72. Golden Couscous Salad

Duration for preparing: 5 mins.
Ready in: 12 mins.
Persons: 4

Required Material:
- 60ml Oil of olive
- 1 medium shallot
- 2.5g ground coriander
- 2.5g turmeric
- 1.25g ground cayenne
- 190g couscous
- 480ml vegetable broth
- Salt
- One yellow bell pepper and one carrot
- 70g apricots
- 40g golden raisins
- 40g cashews
- 225g cooked or (425g) drained chickpeas
- 10g cilantro
- 30ml lemon juice

Instructions:
1. Some oil should be heated in a big pot. It takes around two minutes of stirring to infuse the couscous with the fragrant flavors of the shallot, coriander, turmeric, and cayenne pepper. Avoid letting the ingredients burn together. The broth should be seasoned with salt before being served. Boil, then remove from heat, cover, and set aside for ten minutes to cool slightly before serving.
2. Put the cooked couscous in a large serving bowl. Include a red pepper and a carrot in your list of ingredients along with cashews, chickpeas, apricots, raisins, and cilantro. Give everything a quick toss to combine, and set it aside.
3. Combine the remaining oil with the citrus juice and toss to combine. The salad is ready to be served once the dressing has been poured over the top, and the ingredients have been gently tossed together.

Nutritional breakdown:
Calories: 425, Fat: 18g, Sodium: 636mg, Carbohydrates: 57.6g, Fiber: 9g, Sugars: 18.2g Protein: 11.5g

73. Quinoa Salad with Black Beans And Tomatoes

Duration for preparing: 5 Mins.
Ready in: 20 Mins.
Persons: 4

Required Material:
- 710ml water

- 270g quinoa, well rinsed
- Salt
- 270g cooked or (439g) beans, black
- 80ml red onion
- 60ml parsley
- 4 ripe tomatoes
- 60ml Oil of olive
- 30ml sherry vinegar
- 1g black-pepper

Instructions:
1. Water should be heated to a boil in a large pot after you have added the quinoa and salt. Cover, and cook slowly for about 20 minutes, just below or slightly above the boiling point, or until all the water is absorbed.
2. Cooked quinoa should be put in a very large dish. At this point, you should add the black beans, tomatoes, onions, and parsley.
3. Before adding the sunflower oil, you should mix the olive oil, Apple Cider, pepper, and salt to taste in a small bowl.
4. After you pour the sauce over the salad, give it a good spin to mix everything together.
5. Cover, set away for 20 minutes, and then serve.

Nutritional breakdown:
Calories: 415, Fat: 16g, Sodium: 393mg, Carbohydrates: 56g, Fiber: 13g, Sugars: 5g, Protein: 16g

74. Caesar Salad

Duration for preparing: 10 Mins.
Ready in: 0 Mins.
Persons:1

Required Material:
For The Caesar Salad
- 130g chopped romaine lettuce
- 30g Caesar Dressing
- 1 serving Herbed Croutons or store-bought croutons
- Vegan cheese, grated (optional)

Make It A Meal
- 60g cooked pasta
- 82g canned chickpeas, drained and rinsed
- 30gr additional Caesar Dressing

Instructions:
1. To Prepare The Caesar Salad. Include together insde a big container lettuce, dressing, croutons, and cheese (if using).
2. To Make It A Meal. Add the pasta, chickpeas, and additional dressing. Toss to coat.

Nutritional breakdown:
Calories: 400, Total Fat: 14g, Sodium: 600mg Total Carbohydrates: 57g, Dietary Fiber: 10g, Sugars: 3g, Protein: 14g

75. Classic Potato Salad

Duration for preparing: 10 Mins.
Ready in: 15 Mins.
Persons:4

Required Material:
- 6 potatoes, scrubbed or peeled and chopped
- Pinch salt
- 120ml Creamy Tahini Dressing or vegan mayo
- 2g dried dill (optional)
- 5g Dijon mustard (optional)
- 4 celery stalks
- 2 white - green parts scallions

Instructions:
1. Put the potatoes in a large saucepan, sprinkle them with the salt, and then fill the saucepan with water as long as the potatoes are completely submerged. It is necessary to bring the water to a boil by using a high-heat setting. Cook the potatoes in water that is boiling until they reach the desired consistency, which should be between fifteen and twenty minutes. After the liquid has been drained, set the dish aside to cool.
2. Using a whisk, combine the salad dressing, dill, and brown mustard, if using any of those ingredients. Do this in a large bowl. A mixing dish should be used to incorporate the celery and scallions with the dressing. Include potatoes that have been cooked and left to cool before including them, then toss everything to combine it all.

3. If the leftovers are stored in a container that does not allow air to enter, they may be kept in the refrigerator for up to a week.

Nutritional breakdown:
Calories: 281 kcal, Fat: 8 g, Carbohydrates: 48 g, Fiber: 7 g, Sugar: 4 g, Protein: 7 g, Sodium: 1027 mg

76. Black Bean Taco Salad Bowl

Duration for preparing: 15 mins.
Ready in: 5 mins.
Persons: 3

Required Material:
For the black bean salad
- 397g black beans
- 175g corn kernels, fresh and blanched, or frozen and thawed
- 15g fresh cilantro, or parsley
- Zest and juice of 1 lime
- 2.5g to 5g teaspoons chili powder
- Pinch sea salt
- 225g cherry tomatoes
- 1 red sweet pepper
- Scallions, two

For 1 serving of tortilla chips
- 1 large whole-grain tortilla or wrap
- 5ml Oil of olive
- A dash of salt - oregano - pepper
- Pinch chili powder

For 1 bowl
- 20g fresh greens (lettuce, spinach, or whatever you like
- 150g cooked quinoa, or brown rice, millet, or other whole grain
- 50g chopped avocado, or Guacamole
- 60g Fresh Mango Salsa

Instructions:
How prepare Black Bean Salad
1. Toss All The Ingredients Together In A Large Bowl.

How prepare Tortilla Chips
2. Brush the tortilla with Oil of olive, then sprinkle with salt, pepper, oregano, chili powder, and any other seasonings you like. Slice it into eighths like a Pizza.
3. Transfer the tortilla pieces to a small tray and put inside toaster oven to toast or broil for 3 to 5 mins., till browned. keep an eye on them, as they can go from just barely done to burned very quickly.

To Make The Bowl
4. Lay the greens in the bowl, top with the cooked quinoa, ⅓ of the black bean salad, the avocado, and salsa.

Nutritional breakdown:
Calories: 418, Total fat: 11.5g, Sodium: 331mg, Total carbohydrate: 68g, Dietary fiber: 17g, Sugar: 13g, Protein: 16gù

77. Tuna Caprese Salad

Duration for preparing: 10 mins
Persons: 2

Required Material:
- 2 thinly sliced Roma tomatoes
- 10ml. balsamic vinegar
- 56.7g cubed fresh mozzarella part-skim
- 8 large fresh basil leaves
- 5ml Oil of olive
- 170g fresh tuna steak
- Pepper
- 20ml divided EVO oil

Instructions:
1. Put a big skillet and warm oil (5ml).
2. Once hot, pan-fry tuna for 3 mins. per way. Lay on a dish with a clean paper towel and dab dry. Place in ref to cool for at least an hour.
3. To assemble, layer tomatoes and tuna on a plate.
4. Season with pepper. Sprinkle with basil and mozzarella,
5. Drizzle balsamic vinegar and Oil of olive before serving.

Nutritional breakdown:
Calories: 252, Total Fat: 18 g, Cholesterol: 44 mg, Sodium: 130 mg, Total Carbohydrates: 5 g, Dietary Fiber: 1 g, Sugars: 3 g, Protein: 18 g

Salad Recipes

78. Chopped Salad

Duration for preparing: 15 mins.
Ready in: 0 mins.
Persons: 4

Required Material:
- 177ml Oil of olive
- 59ml wine vinegar
- 10g mustard of Dijon
- 1 garlic
- 8g green onions
- 3g salt
- 0.5g black-pepper
- One head romaine and iceberg lettuce (half of each)
- 274g cooked chickpeas
- 2 ripe tomatoes
- A cucumber
- 2 ribs celery
- A medium carrot
- 60g kalamata olives
- Three red radishes
- 8g parsley
- One ripe Hass avocado

Instructions:
1. If use a blender, food processing equipment, or blender, include all of the necessary ingredients (oil, Apple Cider, brown mustard, garlic, green shallots, and season to taste with spices). Combine everything very well, then set it aside.
2. The two types lettuce should be combined in a large basin and stirred together. At this stage, you should include chickpeas, tomatoes, cucumbers, celery, carrots, olives, and radishes into the meal. Mix in just enough of the dressing so that it completely coats everything. After everything has been mixed together by giving it a little toss, it may be served.

Nutritional breakdown:
Calories: 476, Fat: 42g, Sodium: 641mg Carbohydrates: 22g, Fiber: 9g, Sugar: 6g, Protein: 6g

79. Moroccan Aubergine Salad

Duration for preparing: 30 mins.
Ready in: 15 mins.
Persons: 2

Required Material:
- 4.7ml Oil of olive
- 1 eggplant, diced
- 1.15g ground cumin
- 1g ground ginger
- 0.5g turmeric
- 0.5g ground nutmeg
- Pinch sea salt
- 1 lemon, half zested and juiced, half cut into wedges
- 20g capers
- 10g chopped green olives
- 1 garlic clove, pressed
- Handful fresh mint, finely chopped
- 60g spinach

Instructions:
1. Once you have brought the oil to a to cook slowly in a large skillet fry the eggplant as long as it is soft. After it has grown somewhat softer, which should take approximately 5 minutes, whisk in the nutmeg, cumin, ginger, and turmeric along with a little bit of salt. Cook for around 10 minutes, or till the eggplant has reached the desired degree of tenderness.
2. Add the lemon zest and juice, capers, olives, garlic, and mint. Sauté for another minute or two, to blend the flavors. Put a handful of spinach on each plate, and spoon the eggplant mixture on top.
3. Serve with a wedge of lemon, to squeeze the fresh juice over the greens.
4. The salting of the eggplant will help it to sweat, which will soften it while also removing some of the bitter taste that is naturally present in eggplant. Once dicing the eggplant, sprinkle it with salt and let it sit in a colander for about 30 mins.. Rinse the eggplant to remove the salt, then continue with the recipe as written.

Nutritional breakdown:

Calories: 192 per serving, Total fat: 6.8g, Sodium: 450mg, Total Carbohydrates: 32.2g, Dietary fiber: 15.8g, Sugars: 13.3g, Protein: 6.2g

80. Warm Lentil Salad with Red Wine Vinaigrette

Duration for preparing: 10 mins.
Ready in: 50 mins.
Persons: 4

Required Material:

- 5ml Oil of olive plus 60ml, divided, or 15ml broth or water
- A small onion
- 240ml lentils
- 15g dried basil
- 15g dried oregano
- 15ml red wine or balsamic vinegar (optional)
- 480ml water
- 1 garlic clove
- 60ml red wine vinegar or balsamic vinegar
- 5g sea salt
- One carrot
- 480ml chopped Swiss chard
- 480g torn red leaf lettuce
- 30ml Cheesy Sprinkle

Instructions:

1. After warming 5ml oil in a big skillet, fry the shallot and garlic for five minutes till translucent.
2. Sauté the carrot for three minutes to barely cook it. After tossing in the lentils, basil, and oregano, add balsamic Apple Cider or wine, if using.
3. After adding water, boil it.
4. If cooked gently, lentils should be soft but not falling apart after 20–30 minutes.
5. Mix the red wine Apple Cider, sunflower oil, and salt in a small dish and put aside while the lentils simmer. Drain the lentils and add most of the red wine Apple Cider dressing. Save some dressing.
6. After adding Swiss chard to the saucepan, mix the lentils. Stir the dish for at least 10 minutes on low heat. Mix the lettuce with the dressing.
7. Place lettuce on a dish, then the lentil mixture. Sprinkle a little cheese on the plate and eat it.

Nutritional breakdown:

Calories: 284, Fat: 11g, Sodium: 668mg, Carbohydrates: 35g, Fiber: 15g, Sugar: 4g, Protein: 15g

FISH & SEAFOOD

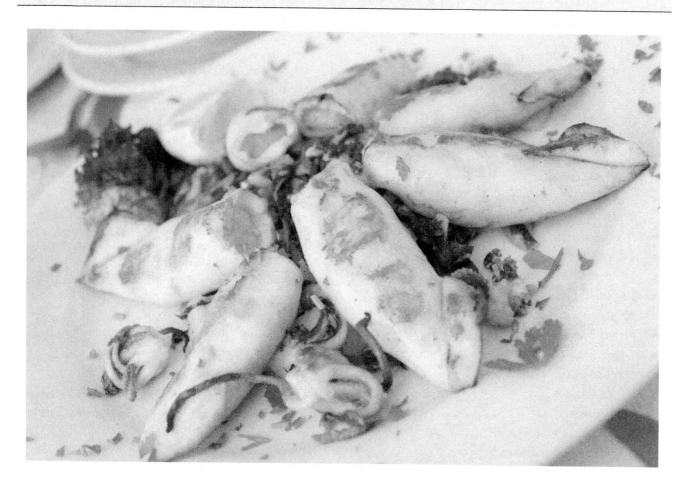

81. Fish Tacos

Duration for preparing: 25 mins.
Persons: 4

Required Material:
- 4 tilapia fillets; cut into medium pieces
- 30 gr coconut flour
- 2 eggs
- 150 gr tapioca starch
- 60 ml sparkling water
- 200 gr cabbage; shredded
- 400 ml coconut oil
- A dash of Sea salt
- Lime wedges for serving
- Black pepper
- Cauliflower tortillas

For the Pico de Gallo:
- 2 tomatoes; chopped
- 30 gr jalapeno; finely chopped
- 90 gr yellow onion; finely chopped
- 30 ml lime juice
- 15 gr cilantro; finely chopped

For the mayo:
- 15 ml Sriracha sauce
- 60 gr homemade mayonnaise
- 10 ml. lime juice

Instructions:
1. Tomatoes, shallot, jalapenos, cilantro, and 2 tablespoons of lime juice should be incorporated in the dish, agitated covered, and refrigerated.
2. Unite mayonnaise, Sriracha, and lime juice on a separate plate. Toss it and put it in the fridge covered.
3. Mix tapioca starch (leave 1/4 for later),

coconut flour, eggs, sea salt, and a few grinds of black pepper in a bowl.
4. Put the remaining tapioca starch in a basin.
5. After patting dry, tapioca pieces should be coated with tapioca starch and dipped in egg mixture.
6. Coconut oil-brushed fish fillets should be cooked in a pan over medium heat. Flip them after one minute and cook for another minute
7. Arrange tortillas on a working surface, divide cabbage on them, add a piece of fish on each, add some of the Pico de Gallo, and top with mayo. Serve with lime wedges.
8. It might seem like a very simple dish, but it's a delicious and fresh!

Nutritional breakdown:
Calories: 648, Fat: 47 g, Carbs: 35g, Fiber: 4g, Protein: 18g

82. Paleo Salmon

Duration for preparing: 30 mins.
Persons: 4

Required Material:
- 6 cabbage leaves; sliced in half
- 4 medium salmon steaks; skinless
- 2 red bell peppers; chopped
- Some oil of coconut
- 1 yellow onion
- A dash of Sea salt
- Black pepper

Instructions:
1. A little amount of water should be added to a pan and warm it. To begin, insert cabbage leaves and blanch them for two minutes. Then you may transfer them from the pan to a plate of ice water.
2. Season each salmon steak with a pinch of sea salt and a few freshly ground grains of black pepper, then wrap it between cabbage leaf halves.
3. Warm a sprinkle's oil in a frying pan; the oil should not smoke. Stirring often, saute the shallot and bell pepper for four minutes.
4. For the baking of the wrapped salmon, put the pan in an oven warmed to 176° degrees

Celsius for around 10–12 minutes. Serve the fish and veggies separately.

Nutritional breakdown:
Calories: 140; Fat: 3g; Fiber: 1g; Carbs: 2g; Protein: 15g

83. Fish Dish

Duration for preparing: 20 mins.
Persons: 4

Required Material:
- 60 g ghee; melted
- 4 halibut fish fillets
- 4 garlic cloves;
- 10 gr parsley; chopped
- Zest and juice from 1 lemon
- 1 lemon; sliced
- A dash of Sea salt
- Black pepper

Instructions:
1. Include garlic with ghee, lemon zest, juice, parsley, sea spices and mix well.
2. Arrange fish in a baking dish, season, drizzle the mix you've made, top with lemon slices, insert in your oven at 220°C and bake for 15 mins..
3. Divide between plates and serve warm.

Nutritional breakdown:
Calories: 250, Fat: 17g, Carbs: 2g, Protein: 23g, Sodium 142mg

84. Salmon Skewers

Duration for preparing: 25 mins.
Persons: 4

Required Material:
- 450 g wild salmon; skinless, boneless, and cubed
- 2 Meyer lemons; sliced
- 60 ml balsamic vinegar
- 60 ml orange juice
- 80 gr Paleo orange marmalade
- A pinch of pink salt
- Black pepper

Instructions:

1. The balsamic vinegar should be heated in a small saucepan. Add the orange juice and marmalade to the saucepan and mix well. Warm for 1 minute, and then turn off the heat.
2. Cubed salmon and lemon slices should be tied together, seasoned with a pinch of salt and pepper, then brushed with half of the Vinegar mixture before being grilled. Then, after preheating the grill, place the skewers on the grill and cook for four minutes each side.
3. Skewers are ready to be served after being brushed with the leftover Vinegar mixture and grilled for one more minute.

Nutritional breakdown:

Calories: 256, Fat: 6g, Carbs: 22g, Protein: 27g

85. Shrimp Dish

Duration for preparing: 20 mins.
Persons: 4

Required Material:

- 1 small red bell pepper; chopped
- 1 small yellow onion; chopped
- 20 shrimp
- 1 garlic clove
- 5 dried red chilies
- 1 small ginger;
- 60 gr coconut aminos
- A dash of Sea salt
- Black pepper
- 28 gr coconut oil
- 30 ml water
- 15 ml lime juice
- 5 ml apple cider vinegar
- 7 gr raw honey
- Handful of cilantro; finely chopped for serving

Instructions:

1. Using a whisk, combine the amino acids, apple cider, honey, water, and lime juice in the dish. Continue whisking until the mixture is smooth.
2. In a skillet that has been already heated with coconut oil, cook the garlic and ginger for two minutes while stirring constantly while keeping the pan moving the whole time.
3. After giving it a toss, continue heating it for another four minutes with the peppers, shallots, and chilies.
4. Cook the shrimp for a further 5 minutes after you have added it, seasoned it to taste with the spices you have made, and stirred in the Apple Cider combination that you have created. When you are ready to serve, divide the mixture out into individual bowls, then dot each with the cilantro.

Nutritional breakdown:

Calories: 157; Fat: 7g; Carbs: 11g; Fiber: 0g; Protein: 5g

86. Grilled Hake

Duration for preparing: 10 mins.
Ready in: 8 mins.
Persons: 4

Required Material:

- 4 hake fillets (500 gr)
- 5 gr salt
- 1 gr ground nutmeg
- 15 gr butter, melted
- 1 gr cayenne pepper

Instructions:

1. Salt, powdered nutmeg, and cayenne pepper have to be mixed together in the basin that you want to make use of for the blending process.
2. First, the spice combination should be worked into the hake fillets, and then the fillets should be coated with butter that has been melted.
3. Get the grill ready to 190 degrees Celsius before you start using it.
4. Put the fish on the grill and allow it to cook for four mins on each side, turning it over once halfway through the cooking process.

Nutritional breakdown:

Calories 165, Fat 4,7 g, Carbs 0,4, g, Protein 30,4 g, Sodium 638 mg

87. Coconut Pollock

Duration for preparing: 10 mins.
Ready in: 15 mins.
Persons: 3

Required Material:
- 312 gr pollock fillet
- 1 bell pepper
- 2 gr smoked paprika
- 2 gr salt
- 170 gr Cheddar cheese, shredded
- 15 gr butter
- 120 ml of coconut milk
- 1 gr turmeric

Instructions:
1. The butter should be melted first, so put it in the pot. Add bell pepper that has been chopped into very little bits. It just takes three minutes to cook.
2. The pollock fillet should be chopped up coarsely. Mix it up with the butter that has been melted.
3. Smoked paprika, salt, and turmeric should be sprinkled over the fish before cooking. Give it a little stir. Cooking slowly, the fish for around five minutes.
4. The coconut milk should be transferred into the other pot. Bring it up to a rolling boil. Pull the pan from the heat and stir in the Cheddar cheese. Carefully combine the cheese with the liquid until it is completely dissolved. Pour the mixture made with the coconut milk over the pollock and bring it to a boil. After that, take the dish away from the heat and let it sit for somewhere in the neighborhood of five minutes.

Nutritional breakdown:
Calories 365, Fat 23, Fiber 1g, Carbs 6g, Protein 32g

88. Spicy Paella

Duration for preparing: 15 mins.
Ready in: 20 mins.
Persons: 3

Required Material:
- 100 g cauliflower, shredded
- 85 g shrimp, peeled
- 85 clams
- 1 garlic clove, peeled
- 1 g sage
- 0,5 g saffron
- 2 g turmeric
- 1 g ground coriander
- 5 g salt
- 15 g butter
- 115 g chicken fillet
- 1 g chili flakes
- 1 g oregano
- 480 ml of water
- 120 ml heavy cream

Instructions:
1. Sage, saffron, turmeric, powdered grains of coriander, oregano, and chili flakes should all be combined in a single bowl before use.
2. Put the butter in the pan and let it to become melted. Include in the shrimp and the clams.
3. Distribute the spice combination over the shellfish and thoroughly combine the two before adding the heavy cream, garlic cloves or lobes, and chicken fillet in very small pieces that have been cut. After thoroughly combining the ingredients, place them in the oven for about five minutes. Incorporate cauliflower and water.
4. Paella should be cooked over medium heat with the cover on for ten minutes.
5. After removing it from the stove and allowing it to rest for ten minutes, paella should be served either hot or warm.

Nutritional breakdown:
Calories 237, Fat 14.8, Fiber 1.4, Carbs 7.2, Protein 18.9

89. Fish Cakes with Greens

Duration for preparing: 10 mins.
Ready in: 5 mins.
Persons: 4

Required Material:
- 227 g salmon fillet
- 113 g cod fillet
- 1 g chives

- 1 g fresh parsley
- 2 g ground coriander
- 2 eggs, beaten
- 16 g almond flour
- 5 g salt
- 15 ml avocado oil

Instructions:
1. The fillets of cod and salmon should be sliced into very small pieces before being placed in the mixing container.
2. Add the eggs, chives, fresh parsley, powdered grains of coriander, almond flour, and salt to the mixture.
3. Using the spoon, thoroughly combine the fish ingredients in the bowl. Form the mixture into cakes of a size that is neither very large nor extremely little.
4. Include some avocado oil inside the frying pan. At this moment the fish cakes that have been made should be roasted for two and a half minutes on each side.
5. If necessary, pat the cooked fish cakes with paper towels to remove excess frying, and then place them on a serving platter.

Nutritional breakdown:
Calories 249, Fat 16.2g, Fiber 1.1g, Carbs 2.2g, Protein 22.6g

90. Fish Bars

Duration for preparing: 10 mins.
Ready in: 15 mins.
Persons:6

Required Material:
- 285 g tilapia fillet
- 60 ml coconut flour
- 2 eggs, whisked
- 5 g salt
- A pinch of ground black pepper
- 85 g Parmesan, grated
- 5 g butter

Instructions:
1. Toss the minced fish into the dish with the other ingredients.
2. Mix in shredded cheese, coconut flour, beaten eggs, salt, black pepper, powdered grains, and a pinch of salt.
3. Use the spoon to thoroughly combine the ingredients. Put a lot of butter in the casserole dish. Distribute the fish mixture evenly in the mold. Use the knife to form bars.
4. Get the oven ready at 180 degrees Celsius.
5. Prepare the fish pieces for 15 minutes, so that the top is golden brown, inserting with a casserole dish in your oven.
6. Put the finished meal chill for at least an hour before serving.

Nutritional breakdown:
Calories 128, Fat 5.8g, Fiber 0.5g, Carbs 1.4g, Protein 17.6g

91. Tuna Pie

Duration for preparing: 15 mins.
Ready in: 40 mins.
Persons:6

Required Material:
- 1 cup cauliflower
- 3 eggs, boiled
- 1 white onion, sliced
- 1 bell pepper
- 240ml heavy cream
- 200g Monterey Jack cheese, shredded
- 14g butter
- 2g ground black pepper
- 0.5g sage
- 5g salt
- 340g tuna
- 5g chives
- 5ml dried dill

Instructions:
1. Prepare a baking tin for the cauliflower and roast it to 185 °C for 15 minutes after warming your oven.
2. Meanwhile, in a mixing bowl, combine the tuna dill, salt, sage, and ground black pepper. Put it to cook for 5 minutes using a skillet. The next step is to pour the mixture into the pie plate. Include white onion, bell pepper and heavy cream.
3. Take the cauliflower out of the oven after it

is done cooking and place it in a food processor. Blend it as long as it is completely smooth.
4. Cut the hard-boiled eggs in lengthwise after peeling them.
5. Evenly coat the tuna mixture with the cauliflower puree. Next, distribute the sliced hard-boiled eggs over the pie and spatter the shredded cheese on top.
6. Bake the pie for 20 minutes set to 185 degrees Celsius. After baking, the pie should be allowed to cool to room temperature before being cut and served.

Nutritional breakdown:
Calories: 379, Protein: 24g, Fat: 28g, Cholesterol: 206mg, Carbohydrates: 6g, Fiber: 1g, Sugar: 3g, Sodium: 630mg

92. Grilled Calamari

Duration for preparing: 15 mins.
Persons: 4

Required Material:
- 907g calamari tentacles and tubes cut into rings
- 28g. parsley;
- 1 lemon; sliced
- Black-pepper
- 1 lime; sliced
- 2 garlic cloves;
- 45ml. lemon juice
- 60ml Oil of olive
- A dash of Sea salt

Instructions:
1. Combine the calamari, parsley, citrus slices, garlic, lemon juice, spices, and oil. Mix all of the ingredients together till they are evenly distributed.
2. Grill the calamari rings on a grill that has been prepared for five minutes before dividing them among several dishes. Some lemons and limes already sliced accompany the dish, and finish it off with an amount of marinade.

Nutritional breakdown:
Calories: 130; Fat: 4g; Fiber: 1g; Carbs: 3g; Protein: 12g, Cholesterol: 240mg, Sodium: 270mg

93. Scallops, Grapes and Spinach Bowls

Duration for preparing: 10 mins.
Ready in: 13 mins.
Persons: 4

Required Material:
- 1 shallot
- 3 garlic cloves
- 355ml chicken stock
- 30g walnuts, toasted and chopped
- 355ml grapes, halved
- 90g spinach
- 15ml avocado oil
- 454g scallops
- A dash of salt

Instructions:
1. Start by putting the oil in a skillet and after warming add the shallot and garlic, give it a swirl, and let it cook for two minutes.
2. After adding the walnuts, grapes, salt, and pepper, continue to simmer; a good cook is needed for three more minutes while stirring constantly.
3. After adding the scallops to the pan, sauté them for two minutes each side and include the spinach. Will be necessary to give everything a good toss and proceed for an additional three minutes, and then serve the mixture in individual bowls. Enjoy!!

Nutritional breakdown:
Calories: 226, Fat: 8g, Cholesterol: 47mg, Sodium: 363mg, Carbohydrates: 17g, Fiber: 2g, Sugar: 11g, Protein: 22g

94. Spanish Mussels

Serving: 4
Duration for preparing: 10 mins.
Ready in: 23 mins.

Required Material:
- 45ml Oil of olive
- 907g mussels, scrubbed

- Pepper to taste
- 710ml canned tomatoes, crushed
- 1 shallot
- 2 garlic cloves
- 473ml low sodium vegetable stock
- 80g cilantro

Instructions:
1. Put the shallot in a skillet and position it overheat. Give it a stir every 30 seconds for three minutes.
2. Include garlic, stock, tomatoes, and pepper, let simmer for ten minutes, please.
3. Incorporate mussels and cilantro together, and proceed to cook with the cover on for another ten minutes.
4. Have fun with it!

Nutritional breakdown:
Calories: 282, Fat: 12g, Cholesterol: 35mg, Sodium: 668mg, Carbohydrates: 21g, Fiber: 3g, Sugar: 7g, Protein: 23g

95. Tilapia Broccoli Platter

Serving: 2
Duration for preparing: 4 mins.
Ready in: 14 mins.

Required Material:
- 170g tilapia, frozen
- 15g almond butter
- 6g garlic
- 5g lemon pepper seasoning
- 100g broccoli florets, fresh

Instructions:
1. Prepare your oven by warming it to 175 degrees Celsius. Include the fish in individual packages made of aluminum foil. Place broccoli in the center of the fish with lemon pepper on top. Seal the packets. Bake for 14 minutes.
2. Put the garlic and almond butter in a bowl, give it a good stir, and set the combination aside as a condiment. Take the sealed package out of the oven and position it on a serving plate. After smearing almond butter over the fish and broccoli, and then savor the meal!

Nutritional breakdown:
Calories: 207; Fat: 9g; Fiber: 4g; Carbs: 7g; Protein: 26g

96. Halibut And Tasty Salsa

Duration for preparing: 25 mins.
Persons: 4

Required Material:
- 4 medium halibut fillets
- 10ml Oil of olive
- A dash of Sea salt
- 20ml lemon juice
- 1 garlic clove;
- Black-pepper
- 2g sweet paprika

For the salsa:
- 30g green onions; chopped
- 135g red bell pepper; chopped
- 16g. oregano
- One small habanero pepper
- A single garlic clove
- 60ml lemon juice

Instructions:
1. Red bell peppers, habanero, green onion, 60 ml lemon juice, 1 garlic clove, oregano, sea salt, and black pepper should be combined in a bowl and stirred well, then stored in the refrigerator for the time being.
2. To make the paprika sauce, incorporate paprika, olive oil, garlic, and twenty milliliters of fresh lemon juice in a big bowl and whip as long as thoroughly combined. Just throw the fish in there, give it a good rubbing, cover the dish, and set it aside for 10 minutes.
3. Cook the fish for 4 minutes each side on a grill pan after having been marinated in the seasonings. The salsa that you cooked beforehand goes well on top of the fish.

Nutritional breakdown:
Calories: 233, Fat: 7g, Cholesterol: 69mg, Sodium: 157mg, Carbohydrates: 8g, Fiber: 2g, Sugar: 4g, Protein: 34g

97. Light Lobster Bisque

Serving: 4
Duration for preparing: 10 mins.
Ready in: 6 mins.

Required Material:
- 236ml diced carrots
- 236ml diced celery
- 822g diced tomatoes
- 2 whole shallots
- 1 clove of garlic
- 14g butter
- 946ml chicken broth, low-sodium
- 5ml dill
- 5ml freshly ground black pepper
- 2.5g paprika
- 4 lobster tails
- 473ml heavy whipping cream

Instructions:
1. In a bowl appropriate for use in the microwave, combine the butter, garlic, and shallots. Prepare in the microwave for 2 to 3 minutes.
2. Throw in some garlic, onions, carrots, celery, and tomatoes into your Instant Pot. Include chicken broth and flavoring.
3. If you want, you may use a knife to remove the meat from the lobster tails before adding them to the Instant Pot. Cover and cook for 4 minutes. Use HIGH pressure. Slowly, over the course of 10 minutes, let the pressure out.
4. Puree to the consistency you want with an immersion blender once ready mix and after incorporating heavy cream. Savor!

Nutritional breakdown:
Calories: 422 kcal, Total fat: 27 g, Cholesterol: 224 mg, Sodium: 840 mg, Total carbohydrates: 24 g, Dietary fiber: 5 g, Sugars: 12 g, Protein: 23 g

98. Thai Pumpkin Seafood Stew

Serving: 4
Duration for preparing: 5 mins.
Ready in: 35 mins.

Required Material:
- 21g fresh galangal
- A can milk of coconut
- A kabocha squash
- 454g shrimp
- 16 thai leaves
- 680g salmon
- 5ml lime, zest
- 15g lemongrass
- 4 garlic cloves
- 726g of each, clams and mussels
- 28g oil of coconut

Instructions:
1. Take a tiny amount of coconut milk, lemongrass, galangal, garlic, and lime leaves to boiling in a little pot. Keep 25 minutes.
2. Put everything in a fine sieve and pour it into a big soup pot.
3. Toss some Kabocha squash into a hot pan with some oil.
4. Add salt and pepper to taste, then sauté for 5 minutes.
5. Combine with coconut mixture.
6. Fish and shrimp should be cooked in oil (4 minutes) before being seasoned with salt and pepper.
7. Unite the mixture with the coconut milk, the clams and mussels. After passing 8 minutes, then sprinkle with basil and serve!

Nutritional breakdown:
Calories: 603 kcal, Total fat: 36 g, Cholesterol: 284 mg, Sodium: 928 mg, Total carbohydrates: 20 g, Dietary fiber: 5 g, Sugars: 5 g, Protein: 50 g

99. Herbal Shrimp Risotto

Serving: 4
Duration for preparing: 10 mins.
Ready in: 8 mins.

Required Material:
- 907g shrimp with their tails removed
- 237ml instant rice
- 473ml vegetable broth
- 1 chopped-up onion
- 227gr chicken breast cut into fine strips
- 59ml lemon juice

- 5g crushed red pepper
- 59ml parsley
- 59ml fresh dill
- 6 pieces chopped-up garlic cloves
- 6g black pepper
- 57g parmesan
- 230g mozzarella cheese

Instructions:
1. Include together the indicated ingredients in your Instant Pot. Should cooked for 8 minutes with the lid locked and the level of pressure at HIGH.
2. Over the course of 10 minutes is necessary permit the tension out gradually. Distribute some cheese on top after popping the lid up. Eat while it is still hot

Nutritional breakdown:
Calories: 553, Total fat: 16 g, Cholesterol: 425 mg, Sodium: 1443 mg, Total carbohydrates: 45 g, Dietary fiber: 2 g, Sugars: 2 g, Protein: 58 g

100. Mackerel and Orange Medley

Serving: 4
Duration for preparing: 10 mins.
Ready in: 10 mins.

Required Material:
- 4 mackerel fillets, skinless and boneless
- 4 spring onion
- 5ml Oil of olive
- 1-inch ginger piece, grated
- Black pepper as needed
- Juice and zest of 1 whole orange
- 240ml low sodium fish stock

Instructions:
1. Black pepper and olive oil should be rubbed into the fillets to season them.
2. In the Instant Pot, combine the chicken stock, orange juice, ginger, orange zest, and onion.
3. After putting in a steamer basket, add the fillets to the pot. Cook for ten minutes with the cover locked in place. Allow the pressure to on its own over the course of ten minutes.
4. The fillets should be distributed among the dishes, and the orange sauce should be drizzled over the fish from the saucepan.
5. Enjoy!

Nutritional breakdown:
Calories: 184, Total fat: 6 g, Cholesterol: 78 mg, Sodium: 112 mg, Total carbohydrates: 6 g, Dietary fiber: 1 g, Sugars: 3 g, Protein: 27 g

BEEF, PORK, POULTRY & LAMB

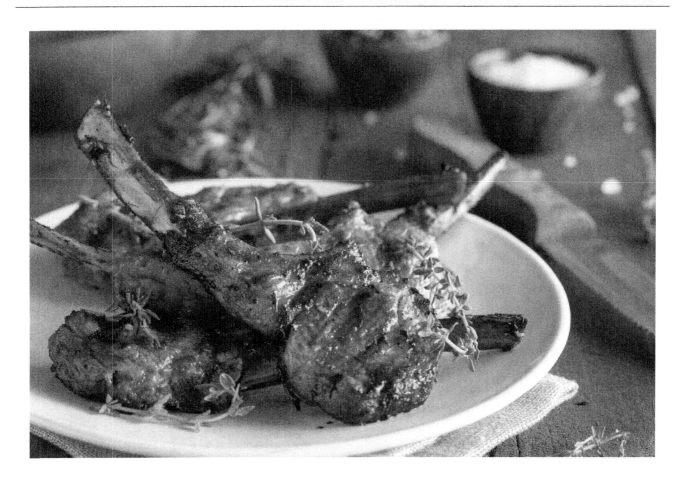

101. Beef Teriyaki

Duration for preparing: 30 mins.
Persons: 4

Required Material:
- 2 green onions; chopped
- 680 g steaks; sliced
- 120 g honey
- 120 ml coconut aminos
- 8 g ginger;
- 8 g tapioca flour
- 15 ml water
- 2 garlic cloves;
- 60 ml pear juice
- Some bacon fat
- 60 ml white wine

Instructions:
1. In a skillet already heated with the bacon grease, cook for two mins after including ginger and garlic, and swirling constantly. Include wine, give it a swirl, then continue cooking as long as it has been absorbed.
2. After adding the honey, amino, and pear juice and stirring, maintain a simmer for a period of 12 minutes.
3. Incorporate the tapioca that has been combined with the water, and then continue to heat it till it thickens.
4. Put the steak pieces in a skillet that has been heated and contains some bacon grease. Brown the steak slices for two minutes on each side.
5. After adding the green onions and half of the newly created sauce, continue cooking for an additional three mins. Serve the meat with

the remaining sauce drizzled on top.

Nutritional breakdown:

Calories: 170; Fat: 3g; Fiber: 2g; Carbs: 2g; Protein: 8g

102. Chicken with Bok Choy

Duration for preparing: 10 mins.
Ready in: 40 mins.
Persons: 4

Required Material:

- 900 g of chicken breast, skinless, boneless, and cubed
- 240 ml bok choy, torn
- 30 ml Oil of olive
- 4 garlic cloves
- A dash of salt, and some freshly powdered grains black pepper
- Cooking spray
- 120 ml pecans, roasted
- 15 ml chives

Instructions:

1. The garlic should be added to hot oil in a skillet and cooked for two minutes.
2. Cook for a further 5 minutes after adding the meat.
3. Toss in the remaining ingredients and slowly cook for 33 minutes.
4. Split it up, and serve it on plates.

Nutritional breakdown:

Calories: 438, Fat: 22g, Saturated Fat: 3g, Cholesterol: 145mg, Sodium: 166mg, Carbs: 8g, Fiber: 4g, Sugar: 2g, Protein: 51g

103. Beef Skillet

Duration for preparing: 50 mins.
Persons: 4

Required Material:

- 454 g beef; ground
- 15 g parsley flakes
- 2 of each: yellow squash and green bell peppers, big tomatoes
- One yellow onion
- Sea salt & pepper (Black)

Instructions:

1. Tomatoes may be cooked on a preheated broiler for 5 minutes, after which they can be peeled and coarsely chopped.
2. Prepare a pan for heating. Put in the onion and meat and shuffle for ten minutes.
3. After adding the tomatoes cook for another 10 minutes and include parsley flakes, black pepper, and a touch of sea salt.
4. Toss in cubes of squash and red bell pepper, and keep on the flame for 10 minutes remembering to stir every now. Serve by dividing among plates.

Nutritional breakdown:

Calories: 291, Fat: 15g, Sodium: 92 mg, Carbs: 13g, Protein: 24g, Sugar: 7g

104. Pork With Pear Salsa

Duration for preparing: 55 mins.
Persons: 4

Required Material:

- 1 yellow onion; chopped
- 1 organic pork tenderloin
- 2 pears; chopped
- 2 garlic cloves;
- 2 g chives; chopped
- 30 g walnuts; chopped
- 45 ml balsamic vinegar
- Black pepper
- 120 ml chicken stock
- 15 ml coconut oil
- 15 ml lemon juice

Instructions:

1. Combine the walnuts, pear, chives, pepper, and lemon juice in a bowl and whisk as long as thoroughly combined.
2. Tenderloin should be browned for 3 min on each side in a hot pan with oil that has been heated.
3. Rotate down the heat, include the onion and garlic, whisk and cook for 2 minutes. Toss in the balsamic vinegar, stock, and pear mixture, and stir. Bake (at 200 °C - 20 mins).
4. 4 minutes have passed and can take away the pork from the oven, let it rest, slice it, and serve it with pear salsa.

Nutritional breakdown:
Calories: 350, Fat: 14g, Sodium: 170 mg, Carbs: 29g, Protein: 27g, Sugar: 17g, Fiber 5g

105. Chicken with Sprouts and Beets

Duration for preparing: 10 mins.
Ready in: 40 mins.
Persons: 4

Required Material:
- 454 g chicken breast
- A dash of salt, and some freshly powdered grains black pepper
- 10 gr (half of each) sweet paprika and coriander
- 1 yellow onion
- 30 ml avocado oil
- Juice of 1 lemon
- 4 garlic cloves
- 100 g Brussels sprouts, trimmed and halved
- 2 beets, peeled and cubed
- 16 g rosemary

Instructions:
1. Throw the onion and garlic into a skillet with the oil and cook them for 5 minutes.
2. Cook for a further 5 minutes after adding the meat.
3. Dip in the remaining ingredients and simmer for 30 minutes.
4. Split it up, and serve it on plates.

Nutritional breakdown:
Calories: 298, Protein: 30g, Fat: 13g, Carbs: 16g, Fiber: 4g, Sugar: 7g, Sodium: 209mg

106. Chicken with Grapes

Duration for preparing: 10 mins.
Ready in: 40 mins.
Persons: 4

Required Material:
- 240 g grapes, halved
- 908 g chicken breast, skinless, boneless, and cubed
- 10 g curry powder
- 30 ml avocado oil
- 4 scallions
- A dash of salt, and some freshly powdered grains black pepper
- 15 g chives

Instructions:
1. In a skillet already heated and with warm oil. include the scallions and cook them for five minutes.
2. After adding the chicken, continue to brown it for another five minutes.
3. Add the other ingredients, give everything a good mix, and then simmer it for half an hour.
4. Parted it up among the plates, and serve it.

Nutritional breakdown:
Calories: 360, Protein: 53g, Fat: 9g, Carbs: 14g, Fiber: 2g, Sugar: 11g, Sodium: 140mg

107. Pork Tenderloin with Carrot Puree

Duration for preparing: 55 mins.
Persons: 4

Required Material:
- 2 sausages; casings removed
- A handful arugula
- Black pepper
- 454 g grass-fed pork tenderloin
- 14 g coconut oil

For the puree:
- 1 sweet potato; chopped
- 3 carrots; chopped
- A dash of Sea salt
- Black pepper
- 15 g curry paste

For the sauce:
- 30 ml balsamic vinegar
- 5 g mustard
- 2 shallots; finely chopped
- Black pepper
- 60 ml EVO oil

Instructions:
1. Open up the pork tenderloin by slicing it horizontally in half but stopping short of the middle.
2. To get a more uniform texture, use a beef

tenderizer.
3. Put the sausage in the center of the pork, then wrap it up around it and knot it with some twine. After that, season it with pepper and set it aside.
4. After preheating an oven-safe pan with the oil from the coconut incorporate the pork roll and cook for three minutes on each side. Then, place the pan in the oven and bake at 175 degrees Celsius (350 degrees Fahrenheit) for twenty-five minutes.
5. In the meanwhile, place the carrots and potatoes in a saucepan, add enough water to cover them, and bring the mixture to a boil. Cook the vegetables for twenty minutes, then drain them and place them in your food processor.
6. To make a puree, give the ingredients a few quick pulses in a food processor, then add a little bit of salt and pepper, give it another whirl, and set it aside in a bowl.
7. Remove the pork roll from the oven, slice it, and then divide it among the plates.
8. Shallots are added to a skillet that has been heated, olive oil is added, and the mixture is stirred while it cooks for ten minutes.
9. After adding the balsamic vinegar, mustard, and pepper, turn off the heat and give the mixture a good toss. Carrot puree should be served with pig pieces, which should then be topped with vinegar sauce and served with arugula on the side

Nutritional breakdown:

Calories: 508, Fat: 34g, Carbs: 24g, Fiber: 4g, Protein: 28g

108. Pork with Strawberry Sauce

Duration for preparing: 45 mins.
Persons: 4

Required Material:
- 1,8 kg pork tenderloin
- 450 g strawberries; sliced
- 10 bacon slices
- A dash of Sea salt
- Black pepper
- 4 garlic cloves;
- 118 ml balsamic vinegar
- 30 ml EVO oil

Instructions:
1. After wrapping the tenderloin in bacon pieces and securing it using toothpicks, season it with salt and pepper.
2. Prepare the tenderloin by placing it on your grill once it has been heated to indirect medium-high heat for thirty minutes.
3. Put the oil in a skillet and heat it over medium-high heat. Add the garlic, toss it around, and let it cook for two minutes.
4. After stirring, bring the mixture to a boil, then add the vinegar and half of the strawberries.
5. Turn the heat down to medium and keep it at a simmer for ten minutes.
6. Stir in the freshly ground black pepper along with the remaining strawberries.
7. Keep cooking the pork over indirect heat while basting it with part of the sauce until the bacon reaches the desired level of crispiness.
8. Place the pork on a cutting board, then let it aside for a few minutes to allow it to cool down. After that, slice the pig and distribute it among the plates. As soon as possible, serve with the strawberry sauce..

Nutritional breakdown:

Calories: 525, Fat: 20g, Carbs: 20g, Fiber: 22g, Protein: 533g

109. Moroccan Lamb

Duration for preparing: 17 mins.
Persons: 4

Required Material:
- 680 g lamb chops
- 14 g ras el hanout
- 5 ml Oil of olive

For the sauce:
- 15 g parsley; chopped
- 4 g mint; chopped
- 3 garlic cloves;
- 12 g lemon zest
- 60 ml Oil of olive
- 1 g smoked paprika
- 1 g red pepper flakes

- 30 ml lemon juice
- A dash of Sea salt
- Black pepper

Instructions:
1. Lamb chops should be seasoned with ras el hanout and oil before being placed on a grill that has been prepared. The chops should be cooked for two minutes each side before being served.
2. In a food processor, combine the parsley, mint, garlic, lemon zest, paprika, pepper flakes, oil, a bit of salt, and ground black pepper. Pulse the mixture extremely thoroughly. Serve the lamb chops with this sauce drizzled over them.

Nutritional breakdown:
Calories: 526, Fat: 46g, Carbs: 1g, Protein: 28g

110. Roasted Lamb

Duration for preparing: 2 hours 40 mins.
Persons: 4

Required Material:
- 15 garlic cloves; peeled
- 6 g onion powder
- 6 lamb shanks
- 4 g cumin powder
- 240 ml water
- 3 g oregano; dried
- 120 ml Oil of olive
- A dash of Sea salt
- Black pepper
- 120 ml lemon juice

Instructions:
1. Put garlic cloves in a roasting pan.
2. Pile the lamb on top of the vegetables, drizzle with half of the oil, and season with a little bit of salt and black pepper.
3. In addition, rub in some cumin and onion powder for added flavor.
4. Put this in the oven at 230 degrees Celsius and roast it for thirty-five minutes.
5. In a dish, combine the remainder of the oil, the water, the lemon juice, and the oregano, and whisk all of the ingredients together very well.
6. After removing the lamb shanks from the oven, pour them with this mixture, toss them so that they are evenly coated, and then return them to the oven to roast at 176 degrees Celsius for two hours and thirty minutes. After dividing the lamb chunks among the dishes, serve.

Nutritional breakdown:
Calories: 868, Fat: 77g, Carbs: 10g, Protein: 34g, Fiber: 1g

111. Beef Casserole

Persons: 6
Duration for preparing: 10 mins.
Ready in: 8 hours

Required Material:
- 340 g pearl onions
- 1,5 kg grass fed beef meat, cubed
- 4 garlic cloves
- 2 sweet potatoes
- 2 celery stalks
- A dash of Sea salt
- Black pepper to taste
- 30 g tomato paste
- 284 g carrot
- 473 g beef broth
- A pinch of thyme dried
- 15 ml coconut oil

Instructions:
1. The beef is browned for two minutes on each side after being placed in a skillet with oil that has been heated, after which it is transferred to a slow cooker.
2. After adding the other ingredients, give everything a good toss, then place the pot in the oven and set the temperature to Low for 8 hours.
3. Enjoy!

Nutritional breakdown: for portion:
Calories 441, Fat 13g, Fiber 5g, Carbs 25g, Protein 56g

112. Grilled Lamb Chops

Persons: 6
Duration for preparing: 10 mins.
Ready in: 10 mins.

Required Material:
- 45 ml coconut aminos
- 60 ml EVO oil
- 8 lamb chops
- A dash of Sea salt
- Black pepper to taste
- 2 garlic cloves
- 30 g ginger
- 3 g parsley leaves

Instructions:
1. Olive oil, coconut amino, garlic, ginger, and parsley are combined in a bowl before being well stirred together.
2. Lamb chops should be seasoned with a pinch of sea salt and freshly ground black pepper to taste before being placed on a grill that has been prepared and adjusted to medium-high temperature. They should be cooked for four minutes each side while being basted with the marinade during the cooking process.
3. After dividing the lamb chops among the platters, serve.
4. Enjoy!

Nutritional breakdown:
Calories: 381 per serving, Fat: 30g, Carbs: 2g, Protein: 25g, Fiber: 0g

113. Lamb Casserole

Persons: 4
Duration for preparing: 2 hours
Ready in: 1 hour

Required Material:
- 1 butternut squash, cubed
- 1,36 kg lamb shoulder
- 4 shallots
- 4 carrots
- 4 tomatoes
- 2 Thai chilies
- 30 ml tomato paste
- 1 cinnamon stick
- 590 ml warm beef broth
- 1 lemongrass stalk, finely chopped
- 5 ml Chinese five spice powder
- 15 ml ginger
- 30 ml coconut aminos
- 22,5 g coconut oil
- 3 garlic cloves
- Black pepper to taste

Instructions:
1. Lamb should be combined in a bowl with coconut aminos, ginger, lemongrass, garlic, and pepper. The mixture should be stirred well, and then it should be covered and stored in the refrigerator for two hours.
2. Bring a saucepan containing the oil to a simmer. Add the lamb that has been marinated, give it a toss, and brown it for three minutes.
3. After adding the tomato paste and the tomatoes, continue to mix for another two minutes.
4. After adding the butternut squash, shallots, Thai chilies, carrots, cinnamon sticks, and five different spices, give the mixture a thorough toss before placing it in your already warmed oven to 325 degrees Fahrenheit for an hour. Divide across plates and serve hot. Enjoy!

Nutritional breakdown:
Calories: 601 per serving, Fat: 30g, Carbs: 34g, Protein: 47g, Fiber: 8g

114. Lamb Chops with Mint Sauce

Persons: 4
Duration for preparing: 15 mins.
Ready in: 20 mins.

Required Material:
- 2 garlic cloves
- 8 lamb chops
- 150 ml EVO oil
- 3 g oregano, finely chopped
- 15 g Dijon mustard
- 6 g lemon zest
- 30 ml white wine vinegar

- 45 g mint
- Black pepper to taste

Instructions:
1. Combine the oregano, garlic, and lemon zest with the olive oil in a bowl and whisk as long as thoroughly combined.
2. Lamb should be rubbed with freshly ground black pepper to taste, and then coated in the newly created mixture.
3. After preheating the grill and adding the lamb chops, allow them to cook for five minutes each side before transferring them to plates.
4. Mustard, vinegar, pepper, and mint are combined in a bowl, and the mixture is then well whisked.
5. A mixture of vinegar and oil should be poured over the lamb chops before serving. Dish up

Nutritional breakdown:
Calories: 765, Fat: 54.3 grams, Carbs: 1.5 grams, Fiber: 2.9 grams, Protein: 63.5 grams

115. Pork with Blueberry Sauce

Persons: 4
Duration for preparing: 10 mins.
Ready in: 30 mins.

Required Material:
- 150 g blueberries
- A pinch of thyme dried
- 900 g pork loin
- 15 ml balsamic vinegar
- A pinch of red chili flakes
- 1 teaspoon ginger powder
- A dash of Sea salt
- 30 ml water

Instructions:
1. Dispose of the pork loin in an ovenproof dish and treat it with a pinch of sea salt and as much black pepper as you want.
2. Blueberries, vinegar, water, thyme, chili flakes, and ginger are combined in a pan that is heated. The pan is then topped with the blueberries.
3. After a thorough stirring and a brief cooking time of five minutes, pour the sauce over the pork loin.
4. Put in the oven at 190 degrees Celsius, and bake for twenty-five minutes.
5. After removing the pork from the oven, let it aside for five minutes, then slice it, portion it out into plates, and serve it with blueberry sauce. Dish up

Nutritional breakdown:
Calories: 572, Fat: 31.7 grams, Carbs: 5.4 grams, Fiber: 0.9 grams, Protein: 62.3 grams

116. Chili Turkey and Peppers

Duration for preparing: 10 mins.
Ready in: 1 hour
Persons: 4

Required Material:
- 30ml avocado oil
- 908g turkey breast, skinless, boneless, and cubed
- 2 color sweet pepper
- Three scallions
- A single red chili
- 1g chili flakes, crushed
- 10g chili powder
- 425g canned tomatoes
- 2 garlic cloves
- 237ml veggie stock
- A dash of salt, and some freshly powdered grains black pepper

Instructions:
1. The oil should be heated in a pan before being added to the pan. The scallions and garlic should then be sautéed for five minutes.
2. After adding the meat, let it brown for five minutes. more.
3. Toss in the bell peppers along with the other ingredients, then simmer for around half an hour.
4. More, portion out into bowls, and enjoy!.

Nutritional breakdown:
Calories: 422 kcal, Carbohydrates: 17 g, Protein: 58 g, Fat: 14 g, Cholesterol: 129 mg, Sodium: 563 mg, Fiber: 5 g, Sugar: 9 g

117. Pulled Pork

Persons: 4
Duration for preparing: 12 hours and 10 mins.
Ready in: 8 hours and 20 mins.

Required Material:
- 118 ml paleo salsa
- 118 ml beef stock
- 118 ml enchilada sauce
- 1,4 kg of organic pork shoulder
- 2 green chilies
- 9 g garlic powder
- 8 g chili powder
- 3 g onion powder
- 2,5 g cumin, ground
- 2 g sweet paprika
- Black pepper to taste

Instructions:
1. Combine the chili powder, chopped onion, and minced garlic in a bowl.
2. Cumin, paprika, and pepper to taste, then whisk everything together after adding the spices.
3. Mix thoroughly, then add the pork, cover, and place in the refrigerator for 12 hours.
4. After transferring the pork to a slow cooker, add the enchilada sauce, stock, salsa, and green chilies. Stir everything together, cover, and simmer on Low for eight hours.
5. Put the pork on a platter, then set it aside to cool off before shredding it.
6. After straining the sauce from the slow cooker into a skillet, bring it to a boil and slowly cook for eight minutes while stirring constantly.
7. After adding the shredded pork and stirring it into the sauce, continue cooking it for another 20 minutes.
8. Distribute across plates and eat hot.!

Nutritional breakdown:
Calories: 1013, Fat: 73 grams, Carbs: 4.3 grams, Fiber: 1.6 grams, Protein: 80.4 grams

118. Turkey with Tomato Asparagus

Duration for preparing: 10 mins.
Ready in: 30 mins.
Persons: 4

Required Material:
- 454g turkey breast, skinless, boneless, and sliced
- 30ml Oil of olive
- 4 scallions
- A dash of salt, and some freshly powdered grains black pepper
- 240ml chicken stock
- 60ml tomato sauce
- 1 bunch asparagus, sliced
- 10ml lemon juice
- 2 garlic cloves
- 15g coriander

Instructions:
1. After heating the oil in a skillet, include the garlic and scallions, and stir-fry the mixture for five minutes.
2. After adding the meat, continue to brown it for another five minutes.
3. Now include the other ingredients, give everything a good toss, and continue cooking it for 20 minutes. Split it up among the plates, and serve it.

Nutritional breakdown:
Calories: 267 kcal, Protein: 29g, Fat: 12g, Carbohydrates: 10g, Fiber: 3g, Sugar: 4g, Sodium: 339mg

119. Beef And Wonderful Gravy

Duration for preparing: 30 mins.
Persons: 4

Required Material:
- 1 egg; whisked
- 15g. mustard
- 15g. tomato paste
- 5g. garlic powder
- 5g. onion powder
- Some coconut oil for cooking
- A pinch of sea A dash of salt, and some freshly powdered grains black pepper
- 680g. beef; ground

For the gravy:
- 10g. parsley; chopped

- 30g. ghee
- 5g. tapioca
- 1 small yellow onion; chopped
- 295ml beef stock
- Black pepper

Instructions:
1. Combine the ground beef with tomato paste, egg, mustard, onion powder, garlic powder, a dash of salt, and a few grinds of black pepper. Mix these ingredients well.
2. Put the ghee in a skillet and allow it to melt over medium heat. Add the onion, give it a toss, and let it simmer for two minutes.
3. After stirring, add the stock, some freshly ground black pepper, and the tapioca that has been combined with water. Continue to cook slowly it till it thickens, then remove it from the fire.
4. Make four patties out of the ground beef mixture. Place the beef patties in a skillet that has been heated with the coconut oil. Cook the burgers for five minutes on each side.
5. After pouring the gravy over the beef patties and topping them with parsley, continue to cook the patties for a few more minutes, and then divide them among plates to serve.

Nutritional breakdown:
Calories: 449, Total fat: 31g, Cholesterol: 177mg, Sodium: 562mg, Total carbohydrate: 5g, Dietary fiber: 0g, Sugar: 1g, Protein: 36g

120. Sheppard's Pie

Duration for preparing: 60 mins.
Persons: 6

Required Material:
- 907g. sweet potatoes; chopped
- 680g. beef; ground
- 475ml beef stock
- 1 onion; chopped
- 2 carrots; chopped
- 2 thyme springs
- 2 bay leaves
- 2 garlic cloves;
- 2 celery stalks; chopped
- 55g ghee
- Bacon fat
- A handful parsley; chopped
- 30g tomato paste
- A dash of Sea salt
- Black pepper

Instructions:
1. After placing the sweet potatoes in a saucepan, fill them with water, bring the pot to a boil, cook the sweet potatoes for twenty minutes, then drain them, allow them to cool, and place them in a bowl.
2. After adding the ghee, season the mashed potatoes with pepper, and salt to taste.
3. Place the beef in a skillet that has been heated over medium-high heat with the bacon grease. Stir the steak occasionally while it cooks for a couple of minutes.
4. After adding the carrots, garlic, onions, celery, stock, tomato paste, bay leaves, thyme springs, more ground black pepper, and a sprinkle of salt, stir the mixture and continue the cook for another ten minutes.
5. To prepare the bottom of a baking dish, remove the bay leaves and thyme, then distribute the meat mixture evenly over the surface.
6. On top, distribute the mashed potatoes evenly before placing the dish inside your already warmed oven to 190 degrees Celsius for around 25 minutes. Wait until the pie has had some time to cool down before slicing it and serving it

Nutritional breakdown:
Calories per serving: 492, Total Fat: 25.3 g, Cholesterol: 103 mg, Sodium: 400 mg, Total Carbohydrates: 36.9 g, Dietary Fiber: 6.1 g, Sugar: 9.8 g, Protein: 30.2 g

SNACKS

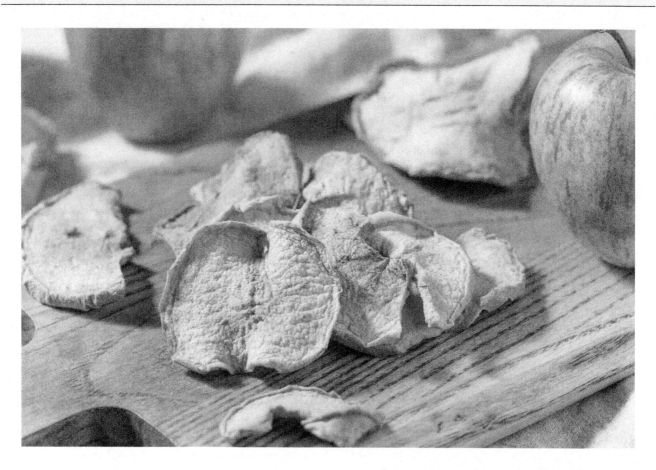

121. Seeds Bowls

Duration for preparing: 10 mins.
Ready in: 15 mins.
Persons: 4

Required Material:
- 120g sunflower seeds
- 80g chia seeds
- 75g pine nuts
- 65g pumpkin seeds
- 15ml coconut oil, melted
- 5ml sweet paprika

Instructions:
1. Put the seeds in an even layer on a cookie sheet that has been coated with parchment paper. Add the oil and paprika, then give everything a good toss before placing it in the oven at a temperature of 200 degrees Celsius for fifteen minutes.
2. To prepare to serve, divide the mixture among bowls.

Nutritional breakdown:
Calories: 388, Fat: 33g, Saturated fat: 6g, Sodium: 4mg, Carbs: 15g, Fiber: 11g, Sugars: 1g, Protein: 15g

122. Almond Artichoke Dip

Duration for preparing: 10 mins.
Ready in: 35 mins.
Persons: 8

Required Material:
- 120ml almond milk
- A pinch of black pepper
- 240ml coconut cream
- 283g canned artichoke hearts, drained

- Four garlic
- 15ml oregano

Instructions:
1. In a saucepan, mix the cream, almond milk, and the other ingredients together, then give the mixture a stir before bringing it to a boil and continuing to cook it for another 35 minutes.
2. Mix the ingredients together with an immersion blender, then place them in separate dishes and use them as a dip for a party.

Nutritional breakdown:
Calories: 111, Fat: 9g, Saturated fat: 5g, Sodium: 84mg, Carbs: 6g, Fiber: 2g, Sugars: 1g, Protein: 3g

123. Snow Peas and Tomato Salsa

Duration for preparing: 10 mins.
Ready in: 0 mins.
Persons: 4

Required Material:
- 240g cherry tomatoes, halved
- 300g snow peas, steamed and cooled
- 15ml lemon juice
- 2 garlic cloves
- 1 avocado, peeled, pitted, and cubed
- 15ml Oil of olive
- 15ml cilantro
- A pinch of cayenne pepper

Instructions:
1. Cherry tomatoes, peas, and the other components should be combined in a dish, then tossed together well before being divided into many smaller bowls and served..

Nutritional breakdown:
Calories: 129, Fat: 10g, Saturated fat: 1g, Sodium: 11mg, Carbs: 11g, Fiber: 6g, Sugars: 2g, Protein: 3g

124. Apple Chips

Duration for preparing: 10 mins.
Ready in: 1 hour
Persons: 4

Required Material:
- Cooking spray
- 2 apples, cored thinly sliced
- 15g cinnamon powder
- A pinch of nutmeg, ground

Instructions:
1. Put the apples in a single layer on a tray that has been prepared with parchment paper, add the other materials, stir, and then bake at 182 degrees Celsius for one hour.
2. Serve as an appetizer by dividing the mixture among bowls.

Nutritional breakdown:
Calories: 64, Sodium: 2mg, Carbs: 17g, Fiber: 4g, Sugars: 11g

125. Dill Cucumber Dip

Duration for preparing: 10 mins.
Ready in: 0 mins.
Persons: 4

Required Material:
- 480ml coconut cream
- 2 cucumbers
- 15ml dill
- 10g thyme
- 10g parsley
- 5g chives
- A pinch of sea A dash of salt, and some freshly powdered grains black pepper

Instructions:
1. Blend the cream with the cucumbers and various other components until smooth, then divide the mixture among dishes, and serve the cucumber salad chilled..

Nutritional breakdown:
Calories: 369, Fat: 35g, Saturated fat: 29g, Sodium: 34mg, Carbs: 13g, Fiber: 3g, Sugars: 5g, Protein: 4g

126. Beans Salsa

Duration for preparing: 15 mins.
Ready in: 0 mins.
Persons: 6

Required Material:
- 480g canned garbanzo and black beans
- 120g cherry tomatoes, cubed
- 1 cucumber, cubed
- 30ml lime juice
- 15ml Oil of olive
- 5 garlic cloves
- 2.5g cumin, ground
- A dash of salt, and some freshly powdered grains black pepper

Instructions:
1. Beans, tomatoes, cucumbers, and all ingredients present on the list should be tossed together in a dish, and then the mixture should be chilled and served as a snack.

Nutritional breakdown:
Calories: 120, Fat: 2g, Sodium: 237mg, Carbs: 21g, Fiber: 6g, Sugars: 3g, Protein: 6g

127. Balsamic Mushrooms Mix

Duration for preparing: 10 mins.
Ready in: 25 mins.
Persons: 6

Required Material:
- 900g brown mushroom caps
- 15ml Oil of olive
- A pinch of sea A dash of salt, and some freshly powdered grains black pepper
- 15ml balsamic vinegar
- 15ml chives
- 5ml sweet paprika

Instructions:
1. Distribute the mushroom caps in a single layer on a tray that has been prepared with paper. Add the oil, salt, and pepper, along with the other components, and give everything a good toss. Bake at 200 degrees C for 25 minutes.
2. Serve by separating the mushroom tops into individual dishes.

Nutritional breakdown:
Calories: 76, Fat: 3g, Sodium: 58mg, Carbs: 12g, Fiber: 4g, Sugars: 6g, Protein: 4g

128. Balsamic Pineapple Bites

Duration for preparing: 10 mins.
Ready in: 20 mins.
Persons: 6

Required Material:
- 397g canned pineapple, cubed
- 2.5g ginger, grated
- 15ml balsamic vinegar
- 2.5g rosemary
- 15ml Oil of olive

Instructions:
1. Combine all elements on the list inside a dish, then toss the mixture, portion it out into bowls, and serve it as a snack.

Nutritional breakdown:
Calories: 78, Fat: 4.6g, Saturated fat: 0.6g, Sodium: 3mg, Carbs: 10g, Fiber: 1g, Sugar: 8g, Protein: 0.6g

129. Parsley Pearl Onions Mix

Duration for preparing: 10 mins.
Ready in: 12 mins.
Persons: 4

Required Material:
- 320g pearl onions, peeled
- Juice of 1 lime
- 15ml Oil of olive
- 6g ginger, grated
- 5g turmeric powder
- 1 small parsley bunch
- A dash of salt, and some freshly powdered grains black pepper

Instructions:
1. Prepare a skillet by heating the oil in the pan. Shake the mixture after adding the pearl onions, lime juice, and the other elements, and then cook it for 12 mins.
2. Offer as a snack by separating the mixture

into separate dishes.

Nutritional breakdown:

Calories: 62, Fat: 3.5g, Carbs: 8g, Protein: 1g, Fiber: 2g, Sugar: 3g, Sodium: 79mg

130. Keto Broccoli Sticks

Duration for preparing: 30 mins.
Persons: 20

Required Material:
- 200g broccoli florets
- 80g panko breadcrumbs
- A drizzle of Oil of olive
- 1 egg
- 40g Italian breadcrumbs
- 6g parsley.
- 40g cheddar cheese, grated
- 30g yellow onion.
- A dash of salt, and some freshly powdered grains black pepper.

Instructions:
1. Broccoli should be added to a pot of water that has been heated; after it has been steamed for one minute, the broccoli should be drained, chopped, and placed in a bowl.
2. After adding the egg, cheddar cheese, panko bread crumbs, and Italian bread crumbs, as well as salt, pepper, and parsley, mix them all together well.
3. Make sticks with your hands using this mixture, and lay them on a baking sheet that has been prepared with olive oil. Bake at 350 degrees for 10 minutes.
4. Put it in the oven at a temperature of 200 degrees Celsius, and bake it for twenty minutes.
5. Prepare for serving by arranging on a dish.

Nutritional breakdown:

Calories: 49, Fat: 2g, Carbs: 4g, Protein: 3g, Fiber: 1g, Sugar: 1g, Sodium: 96mg

131. Nori Snack Rolls

Duration for preparing: 5 mins.
Ready in: 10 mins.
Persons: 4 rolls

Required Material:
- 30g almond, cashew, peanut, or other nut butter
- 4 standard nori sheets
- One mushroom
- 30ml tamari, or soy sauce
- 15gr ginger
- 65g carrots

Instructions:
1. Increase your oven temperature up to 175 degrees C.
2. Combine the nut butter and tamari in a mixing bowl and stir until the mixture is completely smooth and extremely thick. Place a sheet of nori with the rough side facing up and the long way facing you.
3. At the other end of the sheet of nori, spread a very thin layer of the tamari mixture in a line from side to side. At the opposite end, which is the end that is closest to you, arrange the mushroom slices, ginger, and carrots in a line.
4. After rolling the roll toward the tahini mixture, which will act as a binder, fold the veggies inside the nori so that they are enclosed. Repeat to create a total of four rolls.
5. Put the rolls on a baking sheet and bake for eight to ten minutes, or until the edges of the rolls have become slightly browned and crispy. After allowing the rolls to cool for a few minutes, cut each roll into three more manageable pieces.

Nutritional breakdown: (1 roll)

Calories: 80, Fat: 4g, Carbs: 9g, Protein: 3g, Fiber: 2g, Sugar: 2g, Sodium: 321mg

132. Risotto Bites

Duration for preparing: 15 mins.
Ready in: 20 mins.
Persons: 12 bites

Required Material:
- 120ml panko bread crumbs
- 5g paprika
- 5g chipotle in powder
- 355ml cold Green Pea Risotto

- Cooking spray

Instructions:
1. The cookie tray should be prepared with paper after starting your oven (220°C).
2. Combine the paprika, chipotle powder, and panko bread crumbs together on a big dish. Set aside.
3. Form a ball out of two teaspoons of the risotto using your hands.
4. After a light coating in the bread crumbs, transfer the mixture to the baking sheet that has been previously prepared. Continue in this manner to create a total of 12 balls.
5. Cook the risotto bits for 15 to 20 minutes, or until they start to brown, after spraying the tops of them with nonstick frying spray and baking them. After the cookies have had enough time to cool, they should be stored in a single layer in a big container that is airtight (you may add a sheet of paper for a second layer or place them in a plastic freezer bag).

Nutritional breakdown:
Calories: 82, Total fat: 1.6g, Sodium: 127mg, Total carbohydrate: 14.4g, Dietary fiber: 1.6g, Sugars: 0.8g, Protein: 2.4g

133. Marinated Mushroom Wraps

Duration for preparing: 15 mins.
Ready in: 0 mins.
Persons: 2 wraps

Required Material:
- 45ml soy sauce
- 45ml fresh lemon juice
- 22.5ml sesame oil
- 2 portobello mushroom caps
- 1 ripe Hass avocado
- 2 whole-grain flour tortillas
- 480ml fresh baby spinach
- 1 medium red sweet pepper plus one tomato
- A dash of salt, some freshly powdered grains black-pepper

Instructions:
1. To make the soy sauce, mix the soy sauce, 2 tablespoons of lemon juice, and the oil in a medium bowl. Add the portobello strips, give everything a good toss, and then marinate for at least an hour and up to overnight. Remove the liquid from the mushrooms, then put them aside.
2. Combine the mashed avocado and the remaining tablespoon of lemon juice in a bowl.
3. In order to construct the wraps, lay one tortilla on a work surface and sprinkle part of the mashed avocado on top of it. Add a layer of baby spinach leaves to the top of the dish. Arrange strips of the mushrooms that have been soaked in water along with part of the bell pepper strips in the bottom third of each tortilla. To taste, sprinkle the tomato over top along with a pinch of salt and some freshly ground black pepper grains. Roll up firmly, then cut across the diagonally in half.
4. It is now time to serve, so repeat the process with the other components.

Nutritional breakdown:
Calories: 446, Total Fat: 23.6g, Sodium: 1548mg Total Carbohydrates: 47.6g, Dietary Fiber: 13.7g, Sugar: 6.7g, Protein: 13.1g

134. Curried Tofu "Egg Salad" Pitas

Duration for preparing: 15 mins.
Ready in: 0 mins.
Persons: 4 sandwiches

Required Material:
- 450g extra-firm tofu
- 120ml vegan mayonnaise
- 60ml mango chutney
- 10ml mustard (Dijon)
- 15g curry in powder
- 5g salt
- 0.5g cayenne
- 180g carrots
- 2 celery ribs
- 30g onion
- 8 small lettuce leaves
- 4 whole wheat pita bread

Instructions:
1. Tofu should be crumbled and placed in a big dish once it has been prepared. After adding the mayonnaise, chutney, mustard, curry

powder, salt, and cayenne, whisk well as long as everything is evenly distributed and combined.
2. After adding the carrots, celery, and onion, give the mixture a good swirl to integrate everything. Place in the refrigerator for thirty minutes to let the flavors meld together.
3. Place a leaf of lettuce in the bottom of each pita pocket, and then pour some of the tofu mixtures on top of the lettuce before serving.

Nutritional breakdown:
Calories: 456, Total fat: 22g, Sodium: 1177mg, Total carbohydrates: 47g, Dietary fiber: 8g, Sugars: 15g, Protein: 21g

135. Patch Garden Sandwiches

Duration for preparing: 15 mins.
Ready in: 0 mins.
Persons: 4 sandwiches

Required Material:
- 450g extra-firm tofu
- One medium red bell pepper
- 3 green onions
- 30g shelled sunflower seeds
- 120ml vegan mayonnaise
- 2.5g of each salt and celery salt
- A celery rib
- 0.5g black-pepper
- 8 slices whole grain bread
- 4 slices ripe tomato
- Four leaves of lettuce

Instructions:
1. Tofu should be crumbled before being placed in a big basin. Include the seeds together with the bell pepper, celery, and green onions. Mix the mayonnaise, salt, celery salt, and pepper together in a bowl till everything is evenly distributed.
2. If you want, you can toast the bread. Spread the mixture onto the bread so that it is even on all four pieces. Dispose of a slice of tomato, a leaf of lettuce, and the remaining bread on top of each sandwich.
3. Divide the sandwiches in half across the diagonal, and serve.

Nutritional breakdown:
Calories: 454 Total fat: 24.8g, Sodium: 969mg Total Carbohydrates: 39.5g, Dietary Fiber: 8.7g, Sugars: 7.4g, Protein: 21.4g

136. Spinach Garlic Dip

Duration for preparing: 45 mins.
Persons: 6

Required Material:
- 6 bacon slices
- 142g spinach
- 120ml sour cream
- 226g cream cheese, soft
- 10g garlic
- 7g parsley.
- 85g parmesan, grated
- 15ml lemon juice
- A dash of salt, and some freshly powdered grains black pepper.

Instructions:
1. Start by heating a skillet, then add the bacon and fry it until it reaches the desired level of crispiness. After that, remove it to some paper towels to drain the oil, then crumble it and set it aside in a dish.
2. The bacon fat should be heated in the same skillet. Add the spinach, mix it, and cook it for two minutes before transferring it to a bowl.
3. In a separate bowl, combine the cream cheese, garlic, salt, pepper, sour cream, and parsley, and toss all of the ingredients together well.
4. Add bacon and stir again, after adding lemon juice parmesan, and spinach.
5. After dividing the mixture between the ramekins, insert them in your already-heated oven, after placing in the tray (175 degrees Celsius - 25 minutes). Accompany the dip with crackers.

Nutritional breakdown:
Calories: 410, Total Fat: 37g, Cholesterol: 95mg, Sodium: 620mg, Total Carbohydrates: 6g, Dietary Fiber: 1g, Sugar: 2g, Protein: 14g

137. Sesame- Wonton Crisps

Duration for preparing: 10 mins.
Ready in: 10 mins.
Persons: 12 crisps

Required Material:

- 12 Vegan Wonton Wrappers
- 30ml toasted sesame oil
- 12 shiitake mushrooms
- 4 snow peas
- 5ml soy sauce
- 15ml fresh lime juice
- 2.5g brown sugar
- 1 medium carrot
- Toasted sesame seeds or black sesame seeds, if available

Instructions:

1. Adjust the oven's temperature up to 175 degrees C. Prepare a baking sheet by brushing it with oil and setting it aside. After rubbing 15 ml of the sesame oil into the wonton wrappers, put them in a single layer on the baking sheet. Bake for about 5 minutes, or till golden brown and crisp. Set aside to cool. (Another option is to use mini-muffin pans and place the wonton wrappers inside of them to make little cups for the filling. Coat them with sesame oil, then bake them until they are crisp.
2. Warm up the additional olive oil in a big pan. After adding the mushrooms, continue the cook for 3 to 5 minutes, or as long as they have softened. After stirring in the snow peas and the soy sauce, leave on the flame for another thirty seconds, now position aside to cool.
3. Lime juice, sugar, and the remaining 15 milliliters of sesame oil should be mixed together in a big dish. Mix in the carrot and shiitake combination when it has cooled down. Place one heaping teaspoon of the shiitake mixture on top of each wonton crisp. After sprinkling with sesame seeds, place the mixture on a dish so that it may be served.

Nutritional breakdown:

Calories: 60, Total Fat: 4g, Sodium: 80mg, Total Carbohydrates: 5g, Dietary Fiber: 0.5g, Sugar: 0.5g, Protein: 1g

DESSERTS

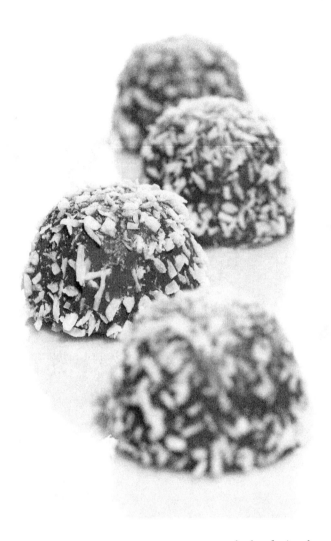

138. Cheesecake

Duration for preparing: 45 mins.

Required Material:

For the crust:
- 57g butter
- 720g coconut, shredded
- Any sweetener you consider appropriate
- 226g cream cheese
- 120ml stevia sweetener
- 120ml maple syrup
- 454g can of pineapple in syrup, crashed or whole, drained
- 60ml whipping cream
- 5 eggs

Instructions:
1. After thoroughly combining all of the ingredients for the crust, give it an even pressing before transferring it to the tint and putting it in the oven for at least ten minutes. Let it cool.
2. Blend the cream cheese, sugars, and pineapple together in a blender till the mixture is smooth and uniform.
3. After gently incorporating the eggs, pour the

mixture into the pan that you have already prepared.
4. Bake for 90 minutes. Take it out of the oven and let it cool.
A helpful hint is that it may be served with extra pineapple on top and/or with whipped cream, as well as any other topping you choose to your preference.

Nutritional breakdown:

Calories: 399, Total Fat: 34.7g, Saturated Fat: 22.1g, Cholesterol: 155mg, Sodium: 237mg, Carbs: 16.3g, Fiber: 2.1g, Sugars: 11.2g, Protein: 8.8g

139. Low-Carb Chocolate Coconut Fat Bombs

Duration for preparing: 95 mins.
Persons: 11-12 balls

Required Material:

- 240g almond butter
- 5 drops vanilla extract (gluten free)
- 20g quality cocoa powder
- 2.5g stevia powder extract
- 3-4 drops of peppermint essential oil (if desired.
- 80g coconut shreds
- 240ml coconut milk

Instructions:

1. To make a double boiler, you may start by placing a glass bowl on top of a saucepan that has a few inches of water in it.
2. In a double boiler, combine all of the ingredients (except for the shredded coconut) to heat them.
3. Include all of the ingredients together and give it a good swirl while you wait for them to come together. When all of the ingredients are evenly distributed across the bowl, take it away from the heat.
4. Put the bowl in the refrigerator for approximately half an hour, or as long as the mixture is sufficiently cold to be rolled into balls.
5. Form the mixture into balls about an inch in diameter, and then roll each ball through the shredded coconut.
6. Put the balls in the refrigerator for one hour after placing them on a dish. Dish and enjoy.
7. If not consumed immediately, store it in the refrigerator.

Nutritional breakdown:

Calories: 238, Total Fat: 22.5g, Saturated Fat: 9.5g, Sodium: 11mg, Carbs: 7.7g, Fiber: 4.7g, Sugars: 1.4g, Protein: 4.4g

140. Crunchy Cherry Chocolate Confections

Duration for preparing: 20 mins. + freezing time
Persons: 30-36 candy cups

Required Material:

- 15ml cherry flavor
- 180g slivered almonds
- 113g. dark chocolate (85 % cocoa solids.
- 120ml organic heavy cream
- 20 drops of liquid stevia

Instructions:

1. Prepare a separate space by chopping the chocolate into very little bits. The next step is to pour the cream into a small saucepan and cook it very slowly till it is really hot, but not boiling. Do not let it boil. Take the pan off the flame.
2. Mix the chocolate that has been cut up into the hot cream. After that, place a lid on it, and let it sit for approximately five minutes.
3. Stir the chocolate and cream mixture together with a spoon for about five minutes, or as long as the mixture is completely smooth and thick.
4. After adding the stevia and the cherry flavoring, whisk the mixture so that it is completely incorporated.
5. After adding the slivered almonds, give the mixture another swirl to be well blended.
6. Pour the mixture in a few tiny candy cups made of paper or foil using a spoon.
7. A night at room temperature or in the refrigerator for a couple of hours, to mature the mixture.

Nutritional breakdown:

Calories: 102, Total Fat: 8.6g, Saturated Fat: 3.9g, Cholesterol: 11mg, Sodium: 7mg, Carbs: 4.2g, Fiber: 1.6g, Sugars: 1.7g, Protein: 1.6g

141. Low-Carb Keto Caramels

Duration for preparing: 15 mins. + refrigeration time
Persons: 10

Required Material:
- 226g butter
- 480ml heavy whipping cream
- 30g stevia powder extract

Instructions:
1. Butter should be melted in a little pot that does not stick, and then it should be allowed to simmer as long as it becomes a light brown hue.
2. The butter should have the cream and stevia added to it, and paddling should continue for approximately two minutes; if keep up the mixture starts to feel sticky and the sauce has thickened.
3. Take the pan off the heat and continue mixing the mixture until it has cooled down a little bit to prevent it from being separated.
4. Fill candy molds with the mixture, then place them in the refrigerator for approximately three to four hours, or until the candy has hardened.

Nutritional breakdown:
Calories: 339, Total Fat: 36g, Saturated Fat: 23g, Cholesterol: 119mg, Sodium: 162mg, Carbs: 4.5g, Sugars: 3g, Protein: 2g

142. Coconut Chocolate Bars

Duration for preparing: 35 mins. + refrigeration time
Persons: 10

Required Material:
- 80ml coconut cream
- 56g coconut oil
- 10g unsweetened cocoa powder
- 80g unsweetened coconut
- 2.5g of Stevia
- 5ml vanilla extract
- 56g butter of cocoa

Instructions:
1. Shredded coconut, coconut cream, 2.5ml of vanilla essence, and 1.25g of stevia should be mixed together well with a spatula. Distribute the coconut flakes on a parchment-lined mini-baking sheet.
2. Form it into a thin, flat rectangle that is 4 inches by 6 inches. You may do this by using a kitchen wrap.
3. Put in the freezer for at least two hours, preferably longer.
4. Take out of the freezer, and divide into 5 individual bars.
5. Getting the chocolate drizzle ready:
6. Coconut oil should be melted in a small pot until it is liquid. To the coconut oil, add the cocoa powder, the rest of the stevia, and the vanilla essence.
7. Let the ingredients amalgamate for 2 minutes, then cool to room temperature while still liquid.
8. Coat the bars uniformly by dipping them in the cocoa mixture and turning them over. The bars' indestructibility is enhanced by being frozen solid. Rearrange the bars on the baking sheet.
9. Once the coating has dried, the bars may be chilled in the fridge.
10. The bars may be stored in the fridge for a firmer texture or at room temperature for a chewier one.
11. When exposed to high temperatures, cacao will melt.

Nutritional breakdown:
Calories: 217, Total Fat: 22.9g, Saturated Fat: 18.4g, Sodium: 4mg, Total Carbs: 4.4g, Fiber: 2.8g, Sugars: 1.1g, Protein: 1.4g

143. Almond-Date Energy Bites

Duration for preparing: 5 mins. • chill time: 15 mins.
Persons: 24 bites

Required Material:
- 200g dates, pitted
- 80g unsweetened shredded coconut
- 60g chia seeds
- 90g ground almonds
- 40g cocoa nibs, or non-dairy chocolate chips

Instructions:
1. Grind all the ingredients together in a food processor until they form a crumbly paste, stopping to scrape down the sides as needed. Soft Medjool dates may be mashed in place of a food processor. However, if you are using tougher baking dates, you will need to soak them before attempting to combine them into a paste.
2. Roll the dough into 24 balls, then set them on a cookie tray with waxed paper. Place in the refrigerator and chill for approximately 15 minutes. Make use of the most forgiving dates you can. The ideal kind of date for this is the Medjool kind. The dry dates you find in the baking section of your grocery store will take forever to puree. If you do decide to use them, it is recommended that you soak them in water for at least an hour before you begin.

Nutritional breakdown:
Calories: 73, Protein: 2 g, Fat: 5 g, Carbs: 7 g, Fiber: 2 g, Sugar: 4 g

144. Keto Chocolate Mug Cake

Duration for preparing: 5 mins.
Ready in: 5 mins.
Persons: 1

Required Material:
- 30g almond flour
- 10g unsweetened cocoa powder
- 30ml heavy cream or unsweetened coconut milk
- 1 large egg, beaten, half for the batter, and more half for topping the mug cake after it is cooked.
- 5g Organic Grade B maple syrup (optional) or 0-calorie sweetener of your choice. Stevia drops would be a great option.

Instructions:
1. In a cup, beat the egg with the cream and maple syrup. Prepare some almond flour and cocoa powder in a cup. Combine all of the ingredients well so that the final product is lump-free and easy to work with.
2. Half of the batter should be spread into the mug's bottom, and the other half should be set aside for the cake's topping. Cook for 30-60 seconds on high power, till the outside is crispy and the inside is still a little uncooked.
3. The cake's center should have the egg used for the batter added to it, and the top should have another tablespoon of beaten eggs, along with the optional cocoa powder and almond flour.
4. Cook for a further 15-30 seconds in the microwave, or until the middle is done.
5. Serve by slicing it up and eating it!

Nutritional breakdown:
Calories: 274, Protein: 12 g, Fat: 23 g, Carbs: 9 g, Fiber: 5 g, Sugar: 1 g

145. Keto Chocolate Chip Muffins

Duration for preparing: 10 mins.
Ready in: 12 mins.
Persons: 12 muffins, 6 servings of 1 muffin each.

Required Material:
- 2 eggs, organic free-range eggs, at room temperature.
- 42g melted butter. Coconut oil, ghee or organic canola oil may be used instead of butter.
- 40g coconut flour
- 80ml unsweetened almond milk
- 5g baking powder
- 10g cocoa powder, unsweetened & 100% cacao.

Instructions:
1. Prepare a muffin pan with 12 paper liners. To use the oven the temperature must be 190 degrees Celsius, and bake the muffins according to the instructions.
2. Eggs and melted butter may be combined with optional vanilla essence. Rest for 5 minutes.
3. The dry components should be added first, followed by the liquids in alternating order.
4. Muffins are done when a toothpick put into the center comes out clean and the muffins are firm to the touch, which usually takes about 12 minutes in a preheated oven.
5. Prepare and savor!

Nutritional breakdown:

Calories: 104, Protein: 4 g, Fat: 9 g, Carbs: 4 g, Fiber: 2 g, Sugar: 1 g

146. Low-Carb, Keto Strawberry Fat Bombs

Duration for preparing: 2 hours
Persons: 15

Required Material:

- 150g strawberries chopped
- 36g powdered erythritol
- 113g cream cheese very soft
- 42g butter very soft

Instructions:

1. In a mixing container, mix together the butter and the cream cheese. Make a paste by mashing everything together with the fork.
2. To prepare the strawberry puree, use a separate bowl. Add the sweetener to the mixture.
3. Either use a spatula to attempt to fold the strawberries into the cream cheese mixture, or alternatively, pour all of the ingredients in a food processor and give it a couple of quick pulses.
4. After the mixture has been piped into the ice cube trays, place them in the freezer for at least two hours. Keep frozen.

Nutritional breakdown:

Calories: 57, Protein: 0.6 g, Fat: 5.7 g, Carbs: 0.6 g, Fiber: 0.2 g, Sugar: 0.3 g

147. Paleo Vegan Peppermint Patties

Duration for preparing: 5 mins.
Persons: 24 cups

Required Material:

- 118ml coconut oil
- 1 serving liquid sweetener of choice
- 120g coconut butter, melted
- 10g peppermint extract
- 170g cocoa chips

Instructions:

1. Prepare a tiny muffin tray with 24 compartments using muffin liners, then put them aside.
2. First, melt 85g of your chocolate chips, then divide them up equally amongst the small muffin pans, making sure that the edges are also coated in chocolate. Refrigerate.
3. If necessary, melt your coconut butter as long as it is completely smooth and creamy. After adding the essence of peppermint, be sure to mix it well.
4. After removing the solid chocolate shells, divide the coconut butter and mint mixture among the chocolates in an equitable manner.
5. To finish off the peppermint patties, melt the second half of the bag of chocolate chips and drizzle it over the top. Refrigerate till firm.

Nutritional breakdown:

Calories: 98, Protein: 1 g, Fat: 10 g, Carbs: 4 g, Fiber: 2 g, Sugar: 1 g

148. Berries and Cherries Bowls

Duration for preparing: 10 mins.
Ready in: 0 mins.
Persons: 4

Required Material:

- 150g strawberries, halved
- 140g blackberries
- 150g cherries, pitted and halved
- 60ml coconut cream
- 60ml stevia
- 5ml vanilla extract

Instructions:

1. Include the berries and cherries together in a dish with the remaining materials, then stir the mixture, portion it out into smaller portions, and serve it chilled.

Nutritional breakdown:

Calories: 83, Total fat: 3.8g, Sodium: 1mg, Total carbohydrates: 14.1g, Dietary fiber: 4g, Sugars: 8g, Protein: 1.2g

149. Cocoa Peach Cream

Duration for preparing: 10 mins.
Ready in: 0 mins.
Persons: 4

Required Material:
- 480ml coconut cream
- 80ml stevia
- 180g cocoa powder
- Zest of 1 lime, grated
- 15ml lime juice
- 2 peaches, pitted and chopped

Instructions:
1. Incorporate the cream, stevia, and cocoa together in a blender, giving it a good whirl after each addition. Pour the mixture into individual serving glasses, and serve it chilled.

Nutritional breakdown:
Calories: 340, Total fat: 32.7g, Sodium: 11mg, Total carbohydrates: 21.5g, Dietary fiber: 8.6g, Sugars: 9.2g, Protein: 4.7g

150. Nuts and Seeds Pudding

Duration for preparing: 10 mins.
Ready in: 20 mins.
Persons: 4

Required Material:
- 340g cauliflower rice
- 60ml coconut cream
- 480ml almond milk
- 5ml vanilla extract
- 36g stevia
- 60g walnuts
- 15g chia seeds
- Cooking spray

Instructions:
1. Match the cauliflower rice with the cream, the almond milk, and the other ingredients in a skillet, and then stir the mixture before bringing it to a simmer and cooking it (20 mins).
2. Separate into bowls, and dish the salad cold.

Nutritional breakdown:
Calories: 151, Total fat: 11.2g, Sodium: 148mg, Total carbohydrates: 9.6g, Dietary fiber: 4g, Sugars: 3.7g, Protein: 5.2g

151. Cashew Fudge

Duration for preparing: 3 hours
Ready in: 0 mins.
Persons: 6

Required Material:
- 80g cashew butter
- 240ml coconut cream
- 120ml cashews, soaked for 8 hours and drained
- 75ml lime juice
- 2.5g lime zest, grated
- 15ml stevia

Instructions:
1. Blend the cashew butter, cream, cashews, juice, and sugar together in a bowl with a whisk till smooth.
2. After lining a muffin pan with parchment paper and placing 1 spoonful of the fudge mixture in each of the tins, place the tray in the freezer for three hours before serving.

Nutritional breakdown:
Calories: 273, Total fat: 25.3g, Sodium: 19mg, Total carbohydrates: 10.6g, Dietary fiber: 1.3g, Sugars: 2.9g, Protein: 5.5g

152. Apple Crumble

Duration for preparing: 20 mins.
Ready in: 25 mins.
Persons: 6

Required Material:
For the filling
- 4 to 5 apples, cored and chopped (about 6 cups
- 120ml unsweetened applesauce, or ¼ cup water
- 20-45g unrefined sugar (coconut, date, sucanat, maple syrup
- 5g ground cinnamon
- Pinch sea salt

For the crumble
- 30g almond butter, or cashew or sunflower seed butter
- 30ml maple syrup
- 180g rolled oats
- 60g walnuts, finely chopped
- 2.5g ground cinnamon
- 20-45g unrefined granular sugar (coconut, date, sucanat)

Instructions:
1. Get your oven ready at 175 degrees C. Coat a square baking dish with sugar, cinnamon, and salt, then add the apples and applesauce. Toss around to mix.
2. Include the nut butter and maple syrup in a medium bowl and stir till combined and smooth. Mix the oats, walnuts, cinnamon, and sugar together as long as well coated. (If you just have a little food processor, chop the oats and walnuts separately and then pulse them together before adding them to the mixture.
3. Toss the apples with the topping and bake until the apples are tender.
4. Cook for 20–25 minutes, or till the fruit is tender and the topping is golden.

Nutritional breakdown:
Calories: 315, Total fat: 12.9g, Sodium: 33mg, Total carbohydrates: 47.7g, Dietary fiber: 7.1g, Sugars: 23.3g, Protein: 6.7g

153. Apricots Cake

Duration for preparing: 10 mins.
Ready in: 30 mins.
Persons: 8

Required Material:
- 180ml stevia
- 240g coconut flour
- 60ml coconut oil, melted
- 120ml almond milk
- 5g baking powder
- 15g flaxseed mixed with 3 tablespoons water
- 2.5ml vanilla extract
- Juice of 1 lime
- 480g apricots

Instructions:
1. After whisking together the flour, coconut oil, and stevia along with the other ingredients, transfer the batter from the bowl into a cake pan that has been prepared with parchment paper.
2. Position in the already-heated oven at 190 degrees Celsius for thirty minutes, then let to cool before slicing and serving.

Nutritional breakdown:
Calories: 240, Protein: 5g, Fat: 12g, Carbohydrates: 32g, Fiber: 10g, Sugar: 5g, Sodium: 125mg

154. Banana Chocolate Cupcakes

Duration for preparing: 20 mins.
Ready in: 20 mins.
Persons: 12 cupcakes

Required Material:
- 3 medium bananas
- 240ml non-dairy milk
- 30g almond butter
- 5ml apple cider vinegar
- 5ml pure vanilla extract
- 150g whole-wheat flour
- 60g rolled oats
- 50g coconut sugar (optional)
- 5g baking powder
- 2.5g baking soda
- 40g unsweetened cocoa powder
- 40g chia seeds, or sesame seeds
- Pinch sea salt
- 40g dark chocolate chips cranberries, or raisins

Instructions:
1. Put the oven on to 175 degrees Celsius before you start. Prepare two muffin trays with six cups each by greasing or lining them with paper muffin cups and applying a light coating of vegetable shortening.
2. Include the bananas, milk, almond butter, vinegar, and vanilla extract into a blender and purée, should obtain completely smooth. Alternately, include all of the ingredients in a large bowl and mix till silky smooth, and creamy.

3. Incorporate flour, oats, sugar (if using), baking powder, baking soda, cocoa powder, chia seeds, salt, and chocolate chips in a separate large basin, and whisk to incorporate all of the ingredients. Combining the dry and wet materials while stirring the mixture as little as possible will provide the best results. Put the mixture into the muffin cups, and bake the muffins for 20 to 25 minutes. Since the cupcakes will be somewhat wet, you should remove them from the oven and allow them to cool completely in the muffin pans before attempting to remove them.

Nutritional breakdown:
Calories: 170, Total Fat: 5g, Sodium: 170mg, Total Carbohydrates: 29g, Dietary Fiber: 6g, Sugar: 8g, Protein: 6g

155. Peach-Mango Crumble (Pressure cooker)

Duration for preparing: 10 mins.
Persons: 4-6

Required Material:
- 720ml of each peach and mango
- 60g unrefined sugar or pure maple syrup, divided
- 120g gluten-free rolled oats
- 60g shredded coconut, sweetened or unsweetened
- 30g coconut oil or vegan margarine

Instructions:
1. Mix the peaches, mangoes, and thirty grams of sugar in a circular baking dish that is between six and seven inches in diameter. Mix the oats, the remaining 30 grams of sugar, and the coconut in a food processor until everything is well combined. Mix thoroughly by pulsing. (If you use maple syrup, you will require less coconut oil. When you add the oil, do so only if the mixture is not adhering together after starting with only the syrup. The oat mixture should be sprinkled all over the fruit combination.
2. Aluminum foil should be used to cover the dish. After placing a trivet in the bottom of the cooking pot of your electric pressure cooker, add a cup or two of water into the pot. The pan should be lowered onto the trivet with either a foil sling or silicone aid handles.
3. High pressure for a period of six minutes. After ensuring that the pressure valve is locked in place and that the lid is closed and locked, choose High Pressure and put the timer on for six minutes.
4. Pressure is let off the hook. As soon as the allotted amount of time for cooking has passed, swiftly release the pressure, taking care not to get your fingers or face too close to the steam release. After the pressure has been completely relieved, the lid should be gently unlocked and taken off.
5. Wait a few minutes for the dish to cool, and then use oven gloves or tongs to gently remove it from the oven. Create individual servings with the scoop..

Nutritional breakdown:
Calories: 279, Total Fat: 11.4g, Sodium: 2mg, Total Carbohydrates: 45.7g, Dietary Fiber: 6.2g, Sugar: 26.9g, Protein: 3.1g

CONCLUSION

The Ketogenic diet is truly life-changing.
The diet improves your overall health and helps you lose extra weight in a matter of days.
The diet will show its multiple benefits even from the beginning, and it will become your new lifestyle really soon.
As soon as you embrace the Ketogenic diet, you will start to live a completely new life.

So, what are you still waiting for? Get started with the Ketogenic diet and learn how to prepare the best and most flavored Ketogenic dishes. Enjoy them all!

CONVERSION MEASUREMENT

Measurement:

1 cup = 24 centilitre (cl) or 240 millilitres (ml)
1 TBSP (tbsp) = 15 millilitres (ml)
1 tsp (tsp) = 5 millilitres (ml)
1 fluid ounce (oz) = 30 millilitres (ml)
1 pound (lb) = 454 grams (gm)
16 ounces = 1 pound
1 millilitre = 1/5 tsp
1 millilitre = 0.03 fluid ounce
1 tsp = 5 millilitres
1 TBSP = 15 millilitres
1 fluid ounce = 30 millilitres
1 fluid cup = 236.6 millilitres
1 quart = 946.4 millilitres
1 litre (1000 millilitres) = 34 fluid ounces
1 litre (1000 millilitres) = 4.2 cups
1 litre (1000 millilitres) = 2.1 fluid pints
1 litre (1000 millilitres) = 1.06 fluid quarts
1 litre (1000 millilitres) = 0.26 gallon
1 gallon = 3.8 litres
1 dash = 1/16 tsp
1 pinch = 1/8 tsp

Abbreviations (Standard English)
Cup = c
Fluid cup = fl c
Fluid ounce = fl oz
Fluid quart = fl qt
Foot = ft
Gallon = gal
Inch = in
Ounce = oz
Pint = pt
Pound = lb
Quart = qt
TBSP = t or tbsp
Tsp = t or tsp